EMOTIONAL HEALING WITH HOMOEOPATHY

Peter Chappell, one of the founding members of the Society of Homoeopaths, has played a key role in the resurgence of homoeopathy over the past 20 years and is currently Director of Overseas Training for the London College of Classical Homoeopathy. He has taught the subject for many years, both in the UK and in Eastern Europe, where he is spearheading homoeopathic training.

Emotional Healing with Homoeopathy

A PRACTICAL GUIDE

Peter Chappell

RSHom

ELEMENT

Shaftesbury, Dorset ● Rockport, Massachusetts
Brisbane, Queensland

© Peter Chappell 1994

First published in Great Britain in 1994 by
Element Books Limited
Shaftesbury, Dorset SP7 8BP

Published in the USA in 1994 by
Element Books, Inc.
PO Box 830, Rockport, MA 01966

Published in Australia in 1994 by
Element Books Limited for
Jacaranda Wiley Limited
33 Park Road, Milton, Brisbane 4064

Reprinted 1995

Cover design by Bridgewater Books
Design by Roger Lightfoot
Typeset by Footnote Graphics, Warminster, Wiltshire
Printed and bound in Great Britain by
Hartnolls Limited, Bodmin, Cornwall

British Library Cataloguing in Publication
data available

Library of Congress Cataloging in Publication
data available

ISBN 1–85230–487–1

Contents

Acknowledgements

I would like to thank all those who have fostered me on my journey in life, especially those who have taught me the most, my parents who gave me my unconscious and those consciousness-making people who include my children Sarah, Elaine and Oliver, my granddaughter Zoe and all the many therapists and friends and lovers I have known, especially Wendy, Jenner and Terry, Alexis, Rosalind, who contributed directly to this book, Melodie, Leigh, Mark, Annie, Julie and all my homoeopathic colleagues and friends. Also my homoeopathic teachers, Thomas Lackenby Maughan, Vasilis Ghegas, George Vithoulkas, Rajan Sankaran and the others who have deeply influenced me. And most of all, my greatest teachers, my patients and students; long have they endured supporting my learning! And to the editors and staff of Element Books for transforming my book, so many thank yous.

Foreword

by Dr Brian Kaplan

No rational person can doubt the fantastic advances made this century by medical science. Potentially fatal diseases including pneumonia, meningitis and tuberculosis are now treated fairly routinely. The discovery of insulin has brought relief to the previously debilitating disease of diabetes. Transplant surgery has given life and mobility to thousands. Demons such as syphilis and Hodgkin's disease have simply been put to the sword.

Nevertheless, many chronic diseases such as eczema, migraine, colitis and arthritis, to name a few, remain very difficult to treat. In spite of this, orthodox medicine, greatly aided by the technological revolution, remains the first choice for most people in the Western world. And notwithstanding great victories in its war against disease, a murmur of dissent is being heard more and more frequently amongst its recipients. Perhaps the reason for this is that as conventional medicine journeys further and further down the electron microscope of scientific discovery, it is losing sight of an ancient healing art. The art of therapeutic listening has sadly been sidelined as the science becomes dominated by deterministic thinking. Wonderful things can be discovered by magnifying diseased tissue, but we are in danger of examining the cells of the tissue and neglecting the patient to whom they belong. By all means, let us look down microscopes at cells, but let us not forget to step back and look at the whole world that these cells occupy. The patient as a whole, personal history, relationships, family, job and position in the community may all have tremendous influence in the causation and perpetuation of disease.

It is ironic that most doctors are all too aware of these influences. No medically trained person would deny that stress and anxiety can lead to a stomach ulcer. And yet the mainstay of the medical treatment of ulcers is by drugs that suppress the secretion of acid in the stomach. Dentists often note the deterioration of gums after a severe shock or disappointment but are trained only to deal with the gums and teeth and therefore often feel powerless to deal with the emotional environment that depressed the immune system and allowed the tissue changes to take place.

For Peter Chappell the psychophysiological changes that allow illnesses to develop and prevent the natural healing ability of the body from curing them, are all important. In this honest and outspoken book, he has drawn not only on his extensive experience as a homoeopathic practitioner but also on his own life and personal exploration with psychotherapy.

It is his view that the susceptibility to disease is usually created by a severe emotional shock to the system. This shock may occur in early childhood, as many a Freudian or Kleinian would concur, or even in utero, since emotional trauma to the mother can affect her physiology profoundly and may be transmitted to the foetus. Of course, as physicians, we may never discover these traumas which are often well hidden and protected, buried in the unconscious mind, all too painful for the patient himself to remember. However, we have a better chance of uncovering these events if we remain silent and allow our patients to speak into a space of compassion and understanding. Peter Chappell has clearly made it his business to make the time for creating such an atmosphere within his practice. The case studies used make for compelling reading. The expert classical homoeopath is much like a detective as he vigilantly searches for clues in his patient's life history that could lead to a successful prescription. These vignettes will surely be described by the medical profession as 'anecdotal evidence' and this is true. The author's theory that deep emotional trauma can produce susceptibility to disease is not scientific since it can be neither proved nor disproved. Nevertheless the stories have an unmistakable ring of authenticity, and most homoeopaths would agree that their remedies, prescribed for the whole person, are capable of producing profound physiological and psychological changes in their patients.

The homoeopathic approach to the patient varies between

two poles. On the one hand the practitioner prescribes for the presenting illness while on the other he listens in silence waiting for the patient to reveal the true centre of his problem. Peter Chappell leans heavily towards the latter approach and this book is a useful contribution to the literature on classical, whole person orientated homoeopathy.

Dr Brian Kaplan MBBCh MFHom
Homoeopathic Physician
February 1994

PART 1

Trauma and suffering

CHAPTER ONE

Trauma, suffering and homoeopathy

This book seeks to provide information about emotional traumas and how they can affect our lives and create our diseases, how they restrict our freedom of expression through suppression and denial of our feelings of fear, anger, grief and loss. These form the basis of what is called disease and by resolving these feelings we can heal our disease.

For many readers the idea of emotional traumas having some effect on diseases may be totally new and in others it may arouse extreme scepticism. However, these are now common ideas in the healing professions.

It may be that we are not even aware of events that have traumatized us in the past. For instance, we may be unaware that an incident which occurred when we were very young might still dramatically affect our behaviour today. This book explains this concept in a clear and straight-forward way. It seeks to awaken your awareness and help empower you to help yourself. It contains enough information to help you heal recent emotional traumas using homoeopathic remedies and illustrates many cases in which this has happened; but it also explains where and when to seek professional help. It details how to bring about truly miraculous cures of 'dis-ease' using homoeopathy in a simple, effective and profound way.

It is aimed at the reader with no prior knowledge of homoeopathy. It can be used for self-help or to guide you to finding professional help for healing. It will also be of interest to student and professional homoeopaths, as it has many new ideas concerning the use of homoeopathy.

Some homoeopaths might criticize me for encouraging self-help, as skilled help is normally more effective. However I also know many people who, given the necessary information, are quite able to help themselves and those close to them. And in many countries where I work, such professional help is simply not available.

So I tread both paths, self-help and professional help, with some trepidation, hoping that you the reader will use your common sense about which is best for you.

HOMOEOPATHY – A BRIEF INTRODUCTION

Homoeopathy has been around about 200 years, and is based on a number of principles and practices that have been tried and tested and found to work consistently for over a century. Samuel Hahnemann, the founder of the system discovered it after meticulous experimentation and observation, and subsequently spent his life refining it.

He found that healing could be based on logical and curative principles. The core principle he discovered is that 'like cures like'. For example, we all know that peeling onions causes itchy and running eyes. These symptoms are typical of hayfever, so hayfever sufferers with these symptoms will be helped by the homoeopathic remedy made from onion. Homoeopaths have found the healing properties of hundreds of substances by trying them out on volunteers, including themselves, and have built up a comprehensive range of remedies that suit most human malfunctions and diseases.

Hahnemann observed that the signs and symptoms of disease are not the disease itself but are reliable indicators of its cure. He discovered that disease is an inner process with rules and logic; it comprises thinking and feeling as well as physical components.

Homoeopathy has been shown to cure thinking, feeling (psychological/emotional) and physical complaints; the principal exceptions are some mechanical injuries needing adjustment (not just spontaneous 'slipped discs' as these can result from inner tension), accidents needing surgery, some life-threatening conditions and some terminal disease states.

Hahnemann also discovered a simple and unique way of preparing the homoeopathic remedies from crude natural substances. Called potentization, it enhances their curative effects whilst removing all side effects. Side effects do not happen in homoeopathy – it is completely safe.

Conventional medical practice generally aims at treating the physical effects of traumas without recognizing or giving attention to the underlying causes, believing in essence that all disease is physical. By diagnosing the physical signs and then opposing and hence denying their effects with drugs, the inner trauma is allowed to grow and possibly fester into a real catastrophe. This is the basic medical approach in diseases such as asthma, eczema, migraines, period problems, arthritis and sore throats.

Homoeopathic remedies by comparison 'mimic' inner traumas; they 'remind' the body to 'unstick and resolve' them so that they can naturally dissolve themselves. In releasing the inner trauma the outer effects (the so-called disease) disappear, cured naturally by the inner healing intelligence (the immune system). This promotes a natural inner process that resolves similar traumas as they occur in the future. For example, if a remedy facilitates a sharp exchange of views and clears the air with beneficial results, a person may see that this is a better way and adopt this approach in future.

NATURAL REMEDIES

Homoeopathic remedies have been selected from thousands of natural substances by a process of clinical elimination over a 200-year period. They now represent a virtually complete set of healing energies appropriate to psychophysical traumatized states and ego-compensations. These energies have, by the complete homoeopathic process, been defined, extracted and stored as pure energy in bottles. They mirror the patterns of traumas built up by the human race since it began.

A WORLDWIDE PERSPECTIVE

Homoeopathy is the second most widely used form of medicine in the world, according to the World Health Organization. Chinese medicine is No. 1, herbalism No. 3 and conventional medicine No. 4. Given that the other systems have been around for thousands of years, this is quite remarkable. Even conventional medicine is basically a continuation of practices established over thousands of years. One man, working largely alone to start with, founded a new medical system that has literally taken the world by storm; and it has been so successful in spite of tremendous opposition because it is so effective. Had homoeopathy met with an intelligent response instead of bigotry, it would probably now be the No. 1 system of medicine everywhere.

MY VIEW

As a practising homoeopath for the last eighteen years, I have seen a great deal of emotional trauma – indeed I have been through a lot of traumas myself. I have put together this book as a result of my inner experiences and my observations in my practice.

I have come to understand that the superficial models of healing that are still common in our culture today, such as the use of drugs and surgery to patch up disease, are often unnecessary and ineffective, even detrimental, and that understanding the cause of the disease, the cause of the emotional reaction which leads to a disease, and its resolution, is a powerfully effective way forward for our well-being today. My belief in this has been confirmed by my teaching experiences with hundreds of doctors, who repeatedly confirm everything I have written here.

Of course, if you have an accident you often need surgery, and surgeons have wonderful skills. And in a well-established pathology which has been left too long, surgical intervention might be appropriate. A new hip is better than a wheelchair. Likewise if you are suffering from a life-threatening illness antibiotics may be the best way to save you. In the acute life crises of the final chronic state, modern medicine is often excellent, but in routine disease its shortcomings are obvious.

Because homoeopathy is a holistic system of curing people my job involves in-depth listening to patients in order to understand their diseases in the context of their lifestyle. As a homoeopath I seek to unite the way of living and the complaints and illnesses in a homoeopathic and holistic synthesis, and finally to follow this with a curative homoeopathic treatment programme.

In consequence, I hear more personal information than most people. I hear thousands upon thousands of life stories, each one of which is unique. Stories of illness and disease are recounted to me along with background feelings of loss, grief, fear, terror, resentment, rejection, lack of caring and much more. Sometimes the stories are of catastrophes, war, violence and abuse. Sometimes I hear about secret police, sometimes about tribal life, sometimes about real poverty. Frequently the patient's dreams also present images and backdrops to the traumas of their recent and distant history. All these are mixed together, woven in patterns that reflect the situation of each individual person in profound yet simple ways that, once seen and understood, can be identified everywhere in the human family worldwide.

HOW THIS BOOK WORKS

In Chapter 2 you will be introduced to some of the basic ideas and examples of emotional traumas and the diseases that follow from them. This will, I hope, help you understand your own inner emotional workings and traumas as well as those of others. This will lead on to Chapter 3, which presents actual case examples and Chapter 4, which looks more deeply at these ideas in action.

The rest of the book concerns itself with how you can deal with these traumas using self-help homoeopathy and professional advice.

CHAPTER TWO

Trauma

SUFFERING

'Life is suffering,' say many of the teachings from India. 'Life is difficult' is the opening sentence of the bestseller *The Road Less Travelled* by Scott Peck. 'Jesus suffered on the cross for us,' it is said. While I am not convinced that we *have* to suffer, I am certain that most people *do* suffer. Suffering occurs in the traumas of growing up, in events like wars and economic recessions, in crises, and in personal or country-wide catastrophes. Bereavement, illness, loss of one's job, loss one's home are all examples of traumatic crises.

In the course of treating people from all corners of the globe, people of all races and all classes, I have heard a lot about suffering. It is, I would say, a universal experience that affects everyone.

TRAUMAS

In this book, I write a lot about the patterns behind suffering, which I call traumas. By this I mean an emotional trauma that comes from feeling hurt. When a particular situation becomes too overwhelming for us to process, the trauma is stored up inside us. I believe that all our dysfunctions ultimately stem from being traumatized and not being able to process it at the time or later.

For example, if someone close to us dies unexpectedly we need to grieve; but if we cannot cry because we have forgotten how, we will start hurting. If we later develop symptoms such as postviral syndrome, chronic weakness, hayfever or headaches, we may well not connect them with the stuck grief. This kind of cause and effect, however, are the 'rule' in understanding health; they follow each other like clockwork. Whenever anyone becomes ill, other than from some obvious contagious disease like measles, it is very useful to question what was going on before it happened – a year or a week or just a minute before.

There are two basic types of trauma: gross and subtle.

Gross trauma

These are overwhelming and sudden traumas. A serious illness in the family, a broken love affair, a rape or violent assault, a sudden divorce, a separation, a death are all common gross traumas where self-help may be appropriate.

In early life incest, violent child abuse, abandonment, adoption, terrifying birth experiences and many more can cause gross traumas in both childhood and adulthood. In these cases professional help might well be needed.

Subtle trauma

These take place subtly and insidiously during growing up, from conception onwards. They can be inflicted by living with a parent who is in trauma and having their trauma reflected onto you, perhaps by cruel, abusive, sad, withdrawn, sarcastic or distant behaviour. A slap, being left to cry, being punished, not being cuddled: if repeated such things can become major traumas for an infant. In the end they cause the child unconsciously to take up a defensive posture to cope with feeling unloved and uncared for.

I see traumas of this sort happening to children all around me in the countries I visit. It is to some extent unavoidable, given that we as parents are ourselves often badly traumatized. These attitudes and actions often seem unimportant to the adults concerned – they are just what their parents did to them – but to the young vulnerable child they can be experienced as an extremely disturbing emotion. These subtle traumas are the root cause of our later inability to process

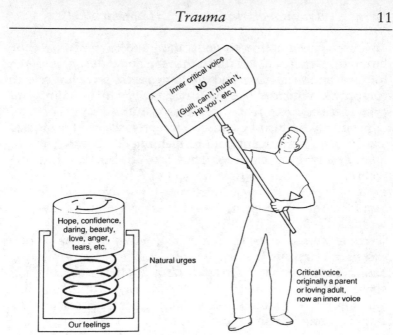

Fig. 1 Subtle trauma leading to the adoption of defensive posture

greater traumas. If we learn not to cry as a child, then as an adult we cannot grieve properly.

There is an even more subtle problem. Some children are born 'sensitive' and need extra loving and caring to thrive. I frequently see sick children whose parents just do not have the ability to be loving enough without further support and training.

A nurse once told me that as a child she laughed a lot. Her loud laughter annoyed her mother so much she was punished. I had already noticed that she was very stiff around her mouth and chin, as if she were permanently trying to hold her mouth under control. She then told me that her son laughed a lot too so I asked how she felt when he laughed. She said, 'I get into such a rage I hit him, I can't help myself.' So the old trauma still dominated her. I asked her why she thought her mother came to hate her laughter and she said that her mother was hit by *her* mother for laughing too. It does not take much imagination to go back a few more generations and see that this is a classic trauma being handed down from generation to generation and to appreciate how powerful it must be. I realized that the nurse's problems were focused on this trauma and could therefore see what remedy to apply to end the line of suffering. Her main complaint, constipation, came from her rigid posture.

Traumas can also be caused by repressed feelings of grief, anger and resentment or tormenting thoughts such as hate, betrayal or rejection. They can arise from crises anywhere: at work, at home or at school. There are many situations in which events can traumatize our lives, including an accident, losing a job, moving house or a holiday that goes wrong.

These things are all happening now, and have been throughout recent history. Modern medicine is now recognizing post-traumatic stress syndrome after wars and personal catastrophes and taking it seriously, with counselling and support. This book is about these personal responses to trauma, whatever the cause.

These two types of trauma, subtle and gross, are really both the same thing. An apparently subtle trauma can be experienced as a gross one by a child in their vulnerable state. The subtle traumas leave the child in a state of lowered self-esteem, less able to cope, so that later gross traumas have an even greater effect, and cannot be processed.

One could postulate that a child brought up with unqualified love and intact feeling release mechanisms (weeping, becoming angry, etc.) would be almost immune to gross overwhelming trauma. They would no doubt feel distressed at the time but when the event was over they would recover by themselves or by seeking help from family and friends.

Such people may exist but they are rare. In the west the social fabric seems to have all but disintegrated into a frivolous, superficial, disconnected TV-hypnotized society. Instead of strong extended families and friendship bonds for life, we see families spread out and connected only by telephones, long motorway journeys and aeroplanes, and friends lost in the constant shifting of our money-centred society. People often have no one to whom they can turn.

Worldwide traumas

The Great Plague wiped out two thirds of the population of many European countries over a 100-year period. American Indians were destroyed in vast numbers by the diseases of the White invaders as well as their guns, until only remnants now survive. These events must have left an indelible mark on the memories of the survivors, which will have been passed on from generation to generation.

One terrible war has spread across the whole world in my lifetime, leaving tremendous devastation from which we are still recovering. We are also faced at this moment with new potential catastrophes: global warming, ozone depletion, pollution of oceans, destruction of wildlife, crises that could wipe out most living things on this planet, ecological catastrophes of unimaginable proportions, traumatic to animals, plants and the earth in unprecedented ways. AIDS threatens whole continents and perhaps others like 'mad cow disease' will do the same. Some say the whole planet is now in deep grief on all levels.

So there is no possibility of an end to worldwide traumas; they are currently epidemic and set to remain so.

THE INNER FEELINGS OF TRAUMA

Traumas usually have an associated set of emotions, including fear, anger, grief/loss and lack of love. In my view these are the primary traumas.

Trauma has stages of occurrence and recovery. There is a trauma 'dynamic' which will vary with each individual according to their self-esteem, previous experiences of trauma, etc. There are some well-established and well-understood patterns of trauma: for example, the work of Elisabeth Kübler Ross on dying, and Alice Miller and others on violence and abuse.

Lack of love seems to me to be the basis of most traumatic feelings, especially isolation, rejection, lack of confidence and poor self-esteem, although fear is also a contributory factor. We all live in a posture which fends off the love by which we are surrounded. As a friend puts it, it is lack of loving that is crucifying us all. The way out is to love, to be loving, not to expect love. In this context love is best defined as kindness, being there for someone, trust, etc., without any sexual connotations.

MAINTAINING NEGATIVE FEELINGS

In my experience fear seems to act as a prison; we are too scared to let in the good around us. We act as if the caring and support available to us is frightening.

Fear of the consequences is often the reason behind holding back the expression of anger. Anger exacerbated by fear can turn inwards and become grief, and despair. These then form the basis for more convoluted sets of emotional trauma states such as depression, guilt, jealousy, loneliness, betrayal, mistrust, violence, abuse, addictive behaviour (alcoholism, drug addiction, smoking, addiction to work or a particular relationship, etc.), all of which can in turn become any illness or disease.

When we become stuck in one state, such as loneliness, hate or depression, we have in effect gone into a closed loop, constantly reaffirming our negative feeling by our reactions to normal living. For example, we feed hatred whenever we restrain our anger rather than express it. If we did not feed our feelings by refuelling them at every possible opportunity, I believe they would die like a fire going out.

Homoeopathic remedies give you the opportunity to let the fire die out or to put it out. If you then take the opportunity to recover, change and enjoy life again, any disease process can be dissolved.

THE DYNAMIC STAGES OF TRAUMA

Denial, fear, terror, grieving, shock, anger, isolation, weeping, separation, rage, loss, joy, acceptance are all feeling stages that can be gone through, often repeatedly, in recovery from trauma, although each individual will get stuck in different places and take different routes according to their recent and underlying history of personal trauma. For example, a person recovering from rape is likely to encounter fear, terror and rage during recovery, whereas a person recovering from a bereavement will focus more on shock, loss, anger and grieving.

This also happens to the perpetrators. People who have commited a serious offence like rape will usually initially deny the offence. Treatment first concentrates on getting them to face the truth. After this may come the recognition of why they did it, perhaps acting out their own victimized state from childhood, and that will require other trauma treatments.

In recovery from bereavement the stages may include denial, anger, guilt, depression, acceptance and finally re-engaging in living positively.

But these are only possibilities. Each individual will tend to 'visit' various feelings according to the many facets of their past and the openings for recovery supporting them. For some the process may include physical illness or emotional pain; for others just a little upset.

The denial stage

When something happens that is overwhelming at the time and nothing is done about it, a common process is to bury it in the tissues and cells of our bodies – to almost deliberately forget about it. This is sometimes the only option, and it may be appropriate at the time. All traumas are like this: what is not processed at the time is blanked out and stored inside. Later the traumas can resurface in many ways as action replays perhaps, or as memories or dreams, or maybe as a disease. At some point a healing intervention may be needed.

Denial and numbing of the trauma come first; after an accident the person classically wanders around saying 'I'm all right' when it is patently obvious they are not. The denial stage can take minutes, hours, days, months, years or even decades. In incest it often persists into adulthood; in an accident it may take minutes, yet it may also take twenty years.

Homoeopathic Arnica is renowned for curing the after-effects of old physical injuries almost by mistake. When a new injury is treated with Arnica, sometimes the after-effect of an old injury, perhaps arthritis, also goes away. Somewhere the body was stuck in an old injury pattern which was released and dissolved by the Arnica. Since the original injury, the muscles would have been in spasm and tension. That requires a feeling or a thought to sustain it, however unconscious, which would have occurred perhaps in a fraction of a second at the time of the original accident.

Such 'blanked out' old emotional traumas lead us to re-enact the events concerned. Violent behaviour and fear of violence, sexual abuse and sexual inhibitions, unnaccountable depression and schizophrenia or any number of delusions, illusions and mental states are almost always based upon real events that we have 'forgotten', because at the time they were too difficult to process.

Denial is a common response to being diagnosed as having a serious disease like cancer. The patient may act as if all is well, even when the surgeon says clearly and sensitively that there is little hope. Denial in this situation can preclude any possibility of recovery, as it is through expression of the fear and rage that inner joy or other resolving feelings can come about. Being stuck in denial stops the healing process.

Denial often occurs even when a patient visits a doctor to have a disease cured. There is usually no idea of the patient's responsibility for causing the disease on the part of either the patient or the doctor, who both carry on as if it's a visitation from the devil or just bad luck. When, as is often the case, the treatment programme offers no cure, just management of the symptoms with increasing side effects and decreasing positive effects, the denial continues.

Medical denial

The signs and symptoms of a disease are not the disease itself; they merely represent the fact that something is wrong. These signs are the positive activity of the immune system doing its best to resolve the problem. Suppression of the signs is like denying that something is wrong and also delays the introduction of a curative strategy. It can damage the immune system by, in effect, telling it that it is wrong. This will often drive the disease process into more severe states.

Papering over the cracks with drugs is a very common way of turning traumas into diseases. A lump in the throat without tears, repeated sighing, headaches and sneezing are all examples of blocked trauma feelings forming into minor signs and symptoms. More severe examples may follow later in life. Denying the trauma is often what passes for health care in our western medical system at present. Even the drug names reflect it: terms like *anti*biotics, pain*killers*, *anti*histamines, *anti*-inflammatory show the ethos of denial which is the basis and substance of drug treatments. Of course drugs may be needed when life is threatened or the disease is too advanced or when good alternatives like homoeopathy are not available. But it is a case of the appropriate use of them. Today they are mostly used inappropriately.

Terror and fear

If terror was experienced in a trauma, then it is likely to resurface in some way.

I was attacked by a strong man wielding a very large knife; the blade was as long as my arm. My immediate instinct was to fight him, but after the first gash I realized that this was stupid and ran. For some weeks afterwards, I was aware of greater fear out on the streets.

Terror and fear can come from attacks, wars, bombs, falls or accidents, even if the person is not physically harmed. Examples are given in the next chapter.

Anger and rage

After a crisis, attack, punishment or annoyance, anger may surface, aimed at the person or people held responsible for the traumatic events. This anger may also be expressed internally as guilt or self-blame: 'If only I had done/not done something.' Rage can be a very appropriate emotion but it is so often repressed because it is regarded as socially unacceptable.

Anger surfaces in bereavement and loss just as much as in violent abuse, and if it is not expressed, depression can result.

Grief

Grief often follows a loss. Weeping is a positive way of releasing it, and is an important part of the healing process.

Recovery

After the negative expressions can come a range of realizations, acceptances and renewed reasons for living and loving. At this point people heal their broken relationships, leave damaging ones, choose new life paths, accept situations, make important decisions or just relax and enjoy what they have.

Here is an example that encapsulates the process, which occurred after taking a homoeopathic remedy. Not all are so dramatic.

> I broke into deep sobbing for no reason, and I felt it was about the old abuse. I was so angry at the abuser and started shouting and crying and then I became scared and thought I was going mad. Then I became so angry with my mother for not protecting me; she must have known, or should have done. I felt guilty at blaming her, but I felt she had let me down, and was never really there for me, especially at crisis times. Later I felt I was going in the wrong direction in my life and that I needed to stay where I was and take stock.

So the person went into grief, then anger, then fear, then anger and blaming, then guilt, then realization and redirection and recovery. This process might all be gone through several times before full recovery.

NATURAL TRAUMA RELEASE

If there is a sympathetic person to listen to you, someone with whom you feel safe, someone to be angry at or a sport or

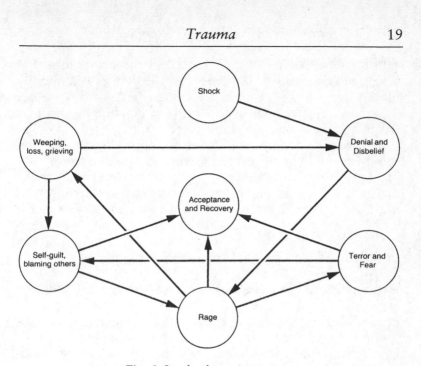

Fig. 2 Stuck places in trauma

activity which will allow your feelings out (football, tennis, golf, squash, swimming, dance, music, theatre, poetry, whatever you like), then you are more likely to resolve the trauma.

Recovery from trauma, either at the time it occurs or later, can be natural. Tears, giggling, talking, swearing, laughing, joking, weeping, sobbing, yawning, sighing and trembling are all ways of recovering from traumas, new or old. Conversely, repeatedly doing any of these things may be a sign of being stuck in a fixed trauma; a constant smile, for example, or frequent giggling or sighing.

Fear can often be released by giggling. Comedians, one type of healer in our culture, invoke giggling frequently through slapstick or embarrassing jokes. Embarrassment is a form of fear, a fear of laughing, the fear of drawing attention to ourselves. After a good laugh we often feel better; something has been released. One man with cancer watched a whole lot of funny videos and laughed himself well. Clearly he knew what worked for him!

Tears can release many forms of loss. All that is needed is a safe place, and for some a cuddle and the acceptance that crying is good and it all comes out. Moody music, moody films, theatre and poetry often act as catalysts for this release.

Sighing releases tension held in the diaphragm and is a frequent release mechanism in some adults.

Swearing, cursing, letting off steam, throwing and kicking things can all help release anger. Hitting a golf or tennis ball, kicking a football and watching sports are also potential release mechanisms. Trembling frequently releases pent-up anger, as indicated by the expression 'He was trembling with anger.'

Inhibition of natural ways of releasing trauma

It is common for the mechanisms by which infants and children release emotional traumas to be blocked. This frequently occurs when the parent, teacher or older sibling acts out programmes of suppressing emotional expression that they learnt as a child themselves. They stop or inhibit the spontaneous releases – giggling, shouting, crying, etc. – often because it upsets them, reminding them of their own unresolved traumas. The expression 'There, there, don't cry' expresses it so well. Usually the 'don't cry' message is accompanied by an implied threat, sometimes a smack or more likely a deliberate distraction ('There there, have a . . .').

Repetition of this suppression will teach the child not to cry (or be angry, dance, be curious, etc.) but in the process it will deny the validity of the child's natural response, denying his or her truth. Systematically applied, this very common approach to parenting blocks off the crying or other reflexes which act as our release mechanisms and makes for the classic 'stiff upper lip' later in life (such people actually have a visibly stiff, strained upper lip).

The crying release is often stopped very early on, before three months or in the first year. It is more common with boys than girls, as in girls tears are generally more acceptable, whilst in boys anger is more tolerated. It is common to find a perverse emotional expression; when one outlet is blocked another acts as a poor and confused substitute. For example girls and women may weep when they are really angry and they can therefore find themselves locked in suppressed anger traumas. This is because they are told not to become angry; it is not socially acceptable. Boys and men can likewise be locked in grief traumas, as the tears will not flow; they will even be angry when in reality they are sad.

Of course these examples are very simplistic, almost stereotypical; many people of both sexes cannot cry or get angry; but they are common traits.

Fear induced inhibition

Fear programming can start with anxious mothers being overcautious about their children being near fire, heights, ponds and other 'dangers', or being overprotective when they are ill, often when there are very reasonable safeguards and very low risks. Safety-consciousness can become an obsession. Through messages like 'keep away', and 'don't do that', children learn not to explore but to act as if there were dreadful danger round every corner. When faced with anything new, they learn to adopt a posture of excessive caution, often restricting their lives to the things they are familiar with.

This form of negative traumatizing is particularly damaging, because fear blocks off the expression of so much else.

THE TRAUMA EMBODIED

When a particular child was excited or upset he was discouraged by his parents; crying was interrupted by kind but distracting comments and excitement reduced to a smile. What the parents did was to shrug their shoulders and pull them together; if you try you will see that it makes it very hard to feel. The child learnt to mimic his parents by a similar shrugging and pulling in of his shoulders and consequently compressed his feelings. Over a period of months and years the child got stuck in this position and grew up thin. He had embodied his trauma, made it part of his way of being. In this way many postural attitudes are transmitted from parent to child and reflect repressed emotional responses and incarcerated traumas.

A baby learnt that when she was upset, food or a dummy were always provided to pacify here. She was given the bottle at every upset, irrespective of real need (a baby's cry can mean feed me, cuddle me, change my nappy, I'm bored, play with me, turn me over, I'm hot/cold, etc.). Now the child, like her parents, eats when she is upset and is growing plump like her parents, who probably had the same upbringing a generation before. (This is a simplification; the infant would initially resist such devices and would have to experience some form of subtle pressure before giving in.)

A boy of fourteen came to see me with eczema. He had been well all his life except for pneumonia once when he was six years old. I noted the sad look in his eyes. I asked him first about his father and he said directly, 'He left when I was five years old.' I understood then that he really felt that he missed his father and that the grief of this probably caused the pneumonia (since grief affects the lungs strongly and chest problems are a frequent result). His eyes told me that he was still suffering, traumatized, in chronic grief.

I needed to make better contact so I asked him about his hobbies; he played football. What position, I asked. Left winger. I asked why the left wing and he said that he seemed to keep 'drifting' to that side. I therefore knew that he felt safer with his left side, which represents the feminine principle (the mother in his case). It is commonly understood that the left side of the body represents feminine qualities (feelings, intuition, being receptive, giving) and the right masculine qualities (physical strength, action, logic) which all of us have, independent of our actual sex.

Basically this boy needed either to see his father very regularly or to find other men to bond to (in the USA they have the 'Buddies' organization especially for this purpose). One of my questions was, 'Why has the eczema come out now?' His mother volunteered that she intuitively felt it was the journey into manhood, acutely felt at this time of puberty, that was causing the stress now. It was bringing the absent father issue poignantly to the fore again.

Trauma, then, had affected this boy profoundly. It coloured his whole perception of life, the sadness flowing out of his eyes. It determined his football position, it determined his illnesses, both acute pneumonia and chronic recurring eczema, and substantially shaped his life. This is true of every trauma that goes unresolved.

INHERITED TENDENCIES

Unresolved traumas and diseases resulting from old traumas often have a history going back to our parents and grandparents. The laughter story on page 11 showed how this can happen. Traumas can in effect be hundreds of years old. You might find it interesting to reflect on your own family patterns of traumas. A good place to start is by talking to the oldest members; from their stories you might find some very revealing patterns. Perhaps you can see their reflection in you.

Some philosophers say that there are no true beginnings. From this standpoint, therefore traumas have always existed and will have been in your family for many generations.

Consider this example. A baby boy is an unwanted fifth child, conceived long after the parents had finished their planned family. He grows up feeling deeply unwanted and his own children are affected, through his re-enactment of his own trauma by abandoning them and through his unfeeling cold nature.

This can go on for generations. 'Third-generation' jealousy is a fairly common problem in my experience.

Familiarity of trauma

When I look at a family together, I am frequently amazed to see the similarity of posture, facial expression, body type, shapes, movements, forms of speech, expressions used and subjects of interest. I find that they seem to match parent to child with extraordinary precision. Traumas can likewise match; they are held inside as memories, thoughts and feelings, and as tensions in muscles, in posture such as a collapsed chest or a stoop, in cells, in all the systems. Traumas show up too as exhaustion, lack of vitality and repressed feelings smouldering inside.

EFFECTS OF TRAUMA IN LIVING

Over- and underreactions

It is common for hurts to be repressed or restricted to some extent because of the programming and blocking off described above. Then the accumulation of little traumas usually grows into one big ball of trauma inside, each new little trauma adding to it until it is finally manifested as disease. Every time a new trauma is then felt, it brings up as a response both the appropriate feeling and all the previous feelings associated with it. An over- or underreaction is the result. Here are some examples of 'overloaded' traumas in action.

If someone were standing on your toe, an appropriate response would be to tell them directly and immediately. 'My toe is hurting because you are standing on it, get off please!'

A traumatized, overreactive response would be: 'Move, you bastard, or I'll smash your face in.' This is a loaded remark, giving no reason, indicating previously repressed anger, a deep trauma, rage and pent-up violence, an aggressive posture.

'Excuse me please, would you mind awfully moving a little, please,' said in a timid quiet voice with a soft smile, likewise giving no reason, would indicate a considerable internalization and repression of anger and a victim posture.

Out of the present

Every old trauma conditions, restricts and overloads our responses to the present moment, keeping us bound into old patterns of behaviour. Instead of responding appropriately to the moment, we bring with us baggage from the past. For example if we hear of the death of a neighbour, we may feel overwhelmed by grief at the memory of the death of our own loved ones.

If we are brought up in fear, we may move very cautiously in everything we do, fear everything new and hate change. If we were subject to violence as children we may feel violent towards our own children, hitting them and overreacting to minor misdemeanours.

Traumas can make us dominate, criticize or abuse others rather than supporting or encouraging them.

These stored up traumas thus shape our everyday responses.

Repetition

When a trauma is stuck inside, it is often repeated time and time again. For example, if a person is stuck in grief, then there are likely to be more situations in their lives which involve grieving. A teenage girl who experienced rejection by her father when he left when she was an infant remained stuck with a idealized version of him. She then tended unconsciously to attract boyfriends who resembled her father, and was rejected. She was not conscious of perpetuating this process but that is what she was doing. Similarly a girl who in the womb was threatened with abortion will pick boyfriends who are threatening and violent.

It is a common experience for many people that when something goes wrong they feel traumatized in a way that reminds them of a similar experience from the past and they relive the pain of the previous event on top of the present one.

In practice it seems that once we have traumas inside us, we attract events which cause a recurrence of the feelings of the previous traumas. I call these 'action replays'.

There is some logic to these recurrences. We are traumatized inside and our deepest inner healing intelligence seeks ways to resolve the problem. Having 'action replays' that remind us of the old traumas can be an active step towards healing ourselves. If through them we receive help that is really appropriate, then it may heal all the previous traumas. Once these are healed, there is no need for further repetition provided there has been an inner resolution and outer changes in behaviour.

So in every crisis in life there are the seeds of our total recovery. That is why it is so important that every crisis be honoured and appreciated for what it is – a total expression of what is wrong.

In homoeopathy we say that a person's signs and symptoms are the body's attempt to display what is wrong. They are not the disease or the trauma but only signs of it. They are, if you like, a mirror of everything to do with the original trauma. So the events of life, especially those which we regard as traumatic and stressful, are the signs and symptoms of 'action replays' of our deepest underlying traumas. By seeing the 'action replays' we can decipher the original traumas. This is a very powerful and practical tool for understanding what has happened in the past. It means that we can work out the past from the present (and vice versa).

This is another aspect of the universal principle that action and reaction are equal and opposite.

Making a career of repeated traumas

Careers can also reflect the 'action replays'. There are many classic examples; the following are all from real life:

- The vet who only found emotional safety with pets as a child;
- The detective who was deceived as a boy;
- The policeman who was beaten as a child;
- The surgeon who as a child had numerous operations;
- The osteopath who was rigidly controlled;
- The prostitute who was sexually abused;
- The lonely child who read a lot and became a librarian;
- The spiritual teacher who was 'disconnected' at birth;
- The girl who first learnt to help her mother to gain approval and now works as a helper.

To varying degrees a primary traumatized state influences the way the person concerned lives; either through their career or in the way they express themselves in their lifestyle. This applies to pop stars and politicians, billionaires as well as office workers. I have known many people who have 'worked on freeing themselves from the past' almost as an obsession, yet still these patterns persist. Our lives are one great big trauma pattern, with the relatively healthy parts mixed in. As a former teacher of mine said, people are a 'loosely connected bunch of ill-assorted attributes'.

Healing these traumas is not, then, an easy process.

The 'action replay' as an addiction

Compulsive and addictive lifestyles reflect the traumatized state and the attempt to hide from it, to deny it and simultaneously to live it out to the full. The term includes relationship addicts who must be in a relationship to feel safe, alcoholics, drug abusers, smokers, compulsive helpers, food bingers, workaholics, compulsive TV watchers – any person whose one core activity dominates their life. These are the large-as-life 'action replays' with one fixed expression dominant as a behaviour. Illness can be seen as another form of addiction in which the behaviour is transformed into disease.

'Action replay' on 'freeze frame'

Some situations may be permanently stressful with no apparent way to change them. These can be called recurring causes of stress that cannot be eliminated. Of course one could argue that all living involves stress, that it is essential to individual and collective progress, and possibly it is. But here we are considering situations where one is trapped in a very stressful situation.

Let us take the case of a man with a well-paid job in a region of high unemployment. Colleagues may say things like, 'You're lucky to have a job here.' He knows jobs are very hard to find, and he is the only breadwinner for a family of five. Yet he hates the job. After many minor illnesses, he catches a cold that goes onto the chest and later he develops pneumonia. This is the only way to get time off, to gain a respite from the stress.

Some jobs just do not suit some people and illness can be an unconscious way of taking time off. Having to work in such a situation can be a repeated trauma and a recurring cause of a sickness.

A sad case of an overwhelming stress is a 'delinquent' child who becomes addicted to drugs and demands more and more money from her doting mother to buy more. The mother, who deeply loves her child, pays up. Later the child relapses into sitting in front of the TV all day, year in, year out. No doctor or psychiatrist can help. The mother cannot talk about it, even to her husband; it is too painful. The father finds consolation and distraction down at the pub with his friends. The mother, stuck in what to her seems an impossible situation, suffering with it deeply and daily, finally contracts cancer and dies.

Such situations may be rare, but lesser ones are very common.

The situation can be corrected, of course. But the person may be completely unaware of it, or too scared to change, or trapped by economic circumstances. Not everyone is ready or willing to make the effort but in the end, some change must be made to bring about a cure. In the final analysis, if the situation is bad enough, they have the option to change consciously or be changed unconsciously by disease or other traumatic events.

The effect of inherited diseases

Inherited diseases, are frequently a major problem for infants. Such diseases often have an effect in infancy and need skilled help.

A history of tuberculosis as a disease trauma in essence means anger stored as sadness in the lungs, and this will lay the foundations for endless chest and respiratory problems, repeating colds, etc., as will any major disease. It is obviously best to try to resolve these before conception; the differences between children conceived before and after the treatment of disease trauma can be quite remarkable. Disease traumas are discussed in more detail in Chapter 3.

COMPLICATIONS IN TRAUMAS

Double binds that restrict healing

A double bind is a situation where the very person who should be able to help you in a crisis is themself involved in it and may be the cause of it.

If your husband dies and you have a best friend to turn to, you can talk it through and recover. But if your best friend then dies it is a different story. After the funeral, you are alone and there is no one you feel is close enough to turn to. That is the double bind and it makes recovery much more difficult.

In divorce, where your spouse may have been your closest confidant, there is no one you can really feel safe to talk things over with. In incest the abuser is often a parent and the other parent may be in silent collusion, so there is no safe place for the distress to be taken. The same can be true of betrayal and many other situations.

The double bind is, then, that the 'traumatizer' is the one the person in trauma would normally turn to for help.

The ironic factor

Trauma tends to stick and be acted out because of one very obvious human instinct. People tend to try to solve a problem by doing the very opposite of what is needed. For example, if you cannot stand your father or mother, using expressions like 'I won't grow up like them', turning away from them and keeping a distance from them makes it more likely that you will turn out like them. To resolve personality problems that stem from your parents, it is better to stay close and 'work through' the irritations inside yourself, otherwise they will grow and solidify. Avoiding the problem will not solve it, it will make it worse. Embracing it is the way through the eye of the needle.

This ironic factor seems perversely to dominate innate human responses to problems. To run away rather than sort them out, to ignore them rather than face them, to buy one's way out rather than be kind, to bury one's head in the sand, are all causes of traumas becoming stuck.

HEALING

Disease as a crisis

Illness and disease can be seen as positive things. They are crises thrown up by our inner needs to resolve old traumas and to change our inner and outer lives. They are crises but not catastrophes.

It helps to know the trauma

Knowing the nature of the underlying trauma can be a great help in knowing how to bring about a resolution, both of the trauma and of its result, the disease. It may also indicate how long the curative process will take and what the signs will be that show that the cure is in progress.

Knowing about traumas – how to live without them, how to recover from them, or how to reduce them – can also be a great aid to parenting and living in general. However, it is possible to help the healing with homoeopathic remedies without knowing the trauma.

Failures of healing

Because of the longevity, the depth and the complexities of the trauma process, superficial healing will often not suffice. Years of treatment, whether conventional or alternative, can be ineffective because it fails to get at the roots of our traumas. Many approaches tend only to scratch the surface. Giving drug-based medicines to treat symptoms is not even scratching the surface; it is merely painting over the cracks or colluding with the denial. It is not in any way attempting to cure.

In my experience, many energetic and vitalizing therapies, including homoeopathy, acupuncture, psychotherapy and osteopathy, fail to get to the roots of illness and traumas because the therapists and patients do not understand or appreciate the depth of the problem or the appropriate resolution. To resolve deep traumas requires accuracy in addressing the core problems, and persistence over months and years in many cases. It also requires the development of a new core process, a new way of functioning, if subsequent traumas are to be processed rather than accumulated again. It needs support in developing ways of expressing anger, fear and grief at the time of the events, rather than incarcerating them. Because all this healing is not easy it is not often achieved.

The healing process

Heal the traumas and the person's natural processes take over and the diseases fade away. The healing treats the traumas, then the body naturally does what it was prevented from doing by the trauma.

My friends in other therapies basically follow this process. Healers do it. Massage therapists do it. Osteopaths do it. Psychotherapists do it in one way or another. This is the universal process we all have to go through to recover from trauma and live our lives to the full.

SUMMARY

In this chapter I have touched upon ideas and concepts that I have noticed and understood about people's lives. These ideas turn up in different guises in all systems seeking to understand the human dilemma and in no way is this more than a cursory glance. Hopefully, however, it is sufficient to allow you to grasp the essential ideas of traumas and the 'stuck energy' nature of illness resulting from traumas.

In the pages that follow you will discover more about traumas and then find the basic information necessary to devise a cure using the homoeopathic way, or how to find other holistic professional help.

CHAPTER THREE

Exploring emotional healing

The cases that follow illustrate through people's actual life stories many of the common traumas that humanity as a whole is living out. Some of these could be helped homoeopathically by the sufferer and some would need a professional helper.

These stories are intended to alert you to the possibilities for trauma that can occur and to give a greater insight into the process. I usually highlight one aspect each time, but invariably the cases overlap and contain many aspects. I have included many different problems but in no way do they cover all known traumas; they are rather a selection representing my own experience.

The sequence of stories starts with grief and loss, as these are most common, then go from conception to the womb, birth, growing up and adult traumas. I have tried to group them as far as possible, but real lives cannot be tidily categorized.

I am also conscious of having simplified some issues and in doing so making the experience seem flat. This is partly to respect the confidence of the people who told me the stories, and partly to keep to simple issues, as in my experience many personal stories boil down to one simple but powerful trauma at their core.

GRIEF TRAUMAS

Death of a spouse

An older woman came to see me. Her husband had recently died and since then she had been experiencing a recurrence of old menopausal symptoms, including terrible hot flushes and other complaints. She had been offered hormone replacement therapy but she knew intuitively that this was not the answer.

A discussion revealed that she had not really cried enough over her loss. The grief was still bottled up, and she was sighing frequently in front of me. What was needed was Ignatia to get her back to good health.

Her trauma was recent grief, with the double bind that she had no one she could talk to, as it was her only close confidant, her husband, who had died. This was compounded by her belief that the 'stiff upper lip' approach was the correct one; she felt that she could not share her sorrow with anyone else. The doctor too had failed to recognize the real problem.

This case is similar to many others. Ignatia was the homoeopathic remedy of choice here as it would facilitate her crying more openly, rather than bottling up the tears at every opportunity, and would allow her menopausal symptoms to fade away.

Repeated disappointment and grief

Sharon was nearly forty and after an unsatisfactory first marriage had settled into a stable relationship with a husband with whom she got on well. She had had mild asthma for many years, and it had recently become much worse.

Sharon had tried to conceive a child with her new husband but could not. Tests showed that her tubes were blocked. At intervals artificial insemination was tried, but nothing happened. At the final attempt before they gave up, it was successful.

However, the previous attempts had led to so much elation followed by disappointment and had brought about such despair and heartbreak that it was not dispelled by the success. Added to this Sharon's father, whom she dearly loved, had died a year earlier. So it was a complex picture of disappointment and grief.

For her increased asthma she needed Ignatia first, to let go of all the stresses of conceiving compounded by the death of her father.

Death at childbirth

A mother died in childbirth while her infant daughter survived. The mother's death was a medical accident, covered
up initially by the doctors in charge but revealed by post
mortem. The father was grief-stricken and felt enraged and
deceived. Unfortunately he was of the 'stiff upper lip' variety
and would not speak about his feelings. For years he held it
all inside. For the newborn child this meant that not only did
she suffer a feeling of abandonment from losing her mother
but she also grew up with a father who was deeply traumatized and 'absent' inside himself – not really available to her
because he was concerned with his own pain.

What will happen when she herself has children? Unless
this double abandonment and grief is resolved, she may well
not feel like having children at all. If she does become
pregnant, she may feel some deep uneasiness about dying
which, if made conscious, might be a fear of dying in childbirth like her mother, compounded by grief about her father/
husband. Or perhaps she will feel too scared to give birth and
need a Caesarean. And what about the child in her womb,
what messages of fear and grief will it pick up there?

The way to help an adult woman in this situation depends
on how the trauma actually happened and on the likelihood
that there is multiple trauma. Such complex traumas often
need sequential treatment, the last one being treated first, so
as to unfold them sequentially backwards in time. The likely
sequence here is grief first and rejection/abandonment
second. The rule in multiple traumas is to take what is 'on
top' first, probably indicated by the 'action replays', and
follow the signs and symptoms as they change into the deeper,
older issue. Even if essentially separate traumas occurred
close in time, they can be separated in recurrence by months
or years.

Of course, in the above case, the history could have been
changed significantly had the father had Ignatia at the time
of the death and had the child also been treated. It is never
too early to treat infants and they respond beautifully to
homoeopathic remedies.

A boy near to death

A boy about nine years old was seriously ill with severe kidney problems. His case had been investigated by many of the best doctors, with no expense being spared. Near to death, the boy was seen in hospital by a homoeopath. It became clear that the parents were in the middle of a protracted and bitter separation and the only reason they were still talking at all was because their child was seriously ill. It was perceived that the child was deeply upset over this separation.

Ignatia, a homoeopathic remedy for disappointment/grief/loss, was given and four days later, to the total amazement of everyone, the child walked into the consulting room, weak but definitely on the mend. The separation was an overwhelming trauma that had been overlooked by the doctors because they are trained to look at physical signs and symptoms of disease, especially when the condition is bad and even more so when death is at hand.

WOMB TRAUMAS

There are many occasions when womb traumas can occur. Two classic times are at conception and at the time the pregnancy becomes a known fact. Examples of these are given below. The state of the parents at conception may be crucial; I suggest that it may be the most important time as it 'sets the tone' for the incoming child.

Trauma in the womb

Two people met on the rebound from two previous relationships. The woman became pregnant. They realized they had made a mistake but stayed together because of the child. Soon they came to hate each other and subconsciously blamed the infant for it. For the child this was very damaging. He grew up as a very angry person without knowing why he felt that way. And as an adult he had nasty-looking red acne to show for it.

Such very early traumas can be unknown to the person concerned, which makes it very difficult to get to grips with them. Parents frequently withhold such information from their children out of guilt or ignorance of the repercussions. However, they can be revealed by recurrences. In some such situations, one might be able to piece together the whole story. Uncles and aunts can often prove useful sources of information.

An unwanted child

I remember a case where a woman wanted the child, her second, but her husband did not. So she became pregnant by him without his knowledge and did not tell him until it was too late. He was furious and wanted a late abortion.

Picture yourself in the womb at the centre of all this. The child probably felt distinctly unwanted, and was born autistic, unable to communicate. He refused to be held by his father for the first two years of his life. He just went into a furious rage, mirroring his father's repressed feelings as well as his own rage, although I doubt if the father saw it. And if he did, what could he do? How could he undo such a trauma in himself and the child?

The idea of the perfect child

It is often said that a newborn child is in a state of perfection. But the state of the parents at conception, their responses to the mother's pregnancy and painful events during the pregnancy will already have provided numerous opportunities to set up traumas before birth. It is thus not possible to have a trauma-free baby, even at birth. Even the mere discussion of an abortion can have an effect.

The idea that events in the womb can affect the child after birth is supported by recent scientific findings. Medical scientists have studied the current and in-the-womb medical records of patients now in their seventies. They have found very reliable correlations between events whilst in the womb and diseases later in life. Extrapolating a little from this research,

I conclude that each organ or body system has a critical short period when it forms and a short crisis at this time can impinge on the growth process. A short upset can affect a person for life, resulting in a weakness in the affected area. A crisis in pregnancy can be the determining factor in the cause of death. The scientists support this thesis by pointing to the fact that forty out of forty-seven levels of cellular division in growth from conception to maturity take place in the womb. It is not surprising, then, that events in the womb represent the most critical phase of life.

Birth is thus far from an ideal state of perfection. Babies will be born traumatized and act out these traumas from their first breath. A beautiful, loving environment is a great thing to aim for in pregnancy and during the first years after birth; it can allow a great deal of healing to take place. Countering this, however, is the reality that virtually all parents are still suspended in their own early trauma and will inevitably be role models for the infant in how to repeat these traumas. Not that this is reason for despair or guilt. I am surrounded by parents of young children (including my daughter and granddaughter) trying successfully to be better parents than their own fathers and mothers.

BIRTH TRAUMAS

It is not generally known that a great variety of traumas can occur at birth and yet in some circles it is seen as the prime trauma time.

Research through regression has shown that there are four stages to the birthing process.

1. *In utero*, initially a state of relative cosmic bliss. We are contained in a warm harmonious liquid, protected from the outside world yet aware of it. Initially we sense our surroundings and later we feel them. So a person stuck in a very sensing way of relating might have a very early *in utero* trauma. In later pregnancy we become increasingly aware of outside influences, knowing what is going on emotionally in our mother, as well as being influenced by the effects of tobacco, alcohol, etc. We begin to feel the effects of the imperfect reality outside.

2. When the uterine contractions start we are violently compressed, under unbearable pressure and strain, and may experience suffocation and a sense of hopelessness.
3. The expulsion stage of the birth process seems cataclysmic, as if the world is being destroyed, or there is a fierce battle, a fight to the death, a death threat, often an experience of dying, of catastrophe.
4. In the final expulsion there is the feeling of liberation, freeing and rebirth, not birth.

Of course medical interferences also come in. At birth forceps will frequently cause a physical trauma and a feeling of intense physical assault, which can last a lifetime. Being stuck in the birthing process can induce suffocation, terror and panic at the thought of dying, which remains for years. In the early moments of life, the separation from the parent can be an overwhelmingly lonely experience. Studies have shown that babies separated even for a few minutes from their mothers directly after birth are less likely to breastfeed successfully and prolonged separation can be the basis for many deep feelings of rejection later in life. Being hung upside down, struck forcibly to 'start' our breathing, being injected, are felt as gross attacks.

A colleague of mind is a practitioner of rebirthing. He tells me that it was originally a Yoga practice for releasing traumas in the body. When this technique was used in western societies it was found that it kept bringing up a wide variety of birth traumas, so it became known as 'rebirthing'. Hundreds of people now practise it and it could be a good way to discover your own birth trauma if your parents will not tell you.

If you are wondering why people believe that what they experience are birthing traumas, here are some of the classic descriptions people have used when talking to me and describing such events.

'It's like a tight band round the head.'
'It feels like a pressure on my head.'
'I dreamt I was in a tunnel' (and claustrophobia in general can have its roots here).
(From a dream) 'It was a wet and hairy place.'
'I dreamt I was in a dark dank place that was very safe too.'

'There was light at the end of the tunnel.'
'When I really feel upset I curl up in a ball' (meaning the womb was the last place that felt really safe).

The graphic detail is surprising and so often it all goes unnoticed. One of my students once read out a whole case to me without realizing any of the subplot messages. Once I started to highlight a few she could not believe how she had missed them.

Medical research

Medical research into suicides has found that the birthing trauma has a strong influence on the type of suicide that can follow. When birth includes lots of drugs the adult may commit suicide by drugs (or, I would conclude, be likely to become a drug abuser). When suffocation occurs in the birth process, suicide by suffocation is the likely form and when mechanical intervention takes place, such as forceps delivery, mechanical means such as hanging are the form of suicide. This fits well with the 'action replay' ideas considered before. All these facts point to the vital importance of birth traumas.

'Action replays' at birth

Reliable clues as to what might go wrong at birth can be deduced from the experience of the mother's or father's own birth, as an 'action replay' is quite likely. Events at previous births should also be considered.

If the father nearly died at birth, so may the first son. If the parent hung on the cord, so may the first child of the next generation. Or if one of the parents refused to feed as a newborn infant, so may the next generation infant of the same sex. 'Action replays' occur again and again in my experience, often with incredible accuracy and consequences. How this process works is hard to understand but my own and my patients' bitter experience has shown it to be a reliable rule and a common process.

So in birthing, old traumas relating to the events of the

birth of the mother and/or father can resurface. It is also likely to restimulate any of the birth traumas of the birth attendants, and this is as good a reason as any for having a home birth.

The birth place

From my own experiences of birth, and from the hundreds of birthing stories I have heard, my deep conviction is that most births, especially the first, should be at home with the *least possible medical intervention*.

Just for a moment imagine that the doctors and midwives at your birth were born in terror although they are not aware of the fact. Imagine, too, that they were all trained in medical school and have seen dramatic live examples of all the things that can go wrong. Imagine that their minds are full of these things and remember the adage 'thought is creative'. As soon as anything seems to be going wrong, up pop all those fears related to extreme complications. Imagine, too, their hidden agendas, the need to protect their careers and to satisfy legal requirements, codes of good hospital practice, etc. There are all these traumas and fears around when what the mother needs is calm, reassurance, peace and loving support.

This is why I recommend minimizing their numbers, unless you are sure they have sorted out their own traumas.

Mechanical birth traumas

Cutting the cord too early can be a trauma and it may not be necessary. My second daughter was born at home with the cord around her neck. Considering that my first daughter died hung on the cord, under full hospital care, I could have panicked. But I stayed calm and as the midwife reached hastily for the cutters I suggested that she gently pull the cord over the head, as there should be plenty inside still. She did this and the birth proceeded naturally.

Episiotomy involves cutting the perineum rather than allowing it to stretch naturally or tear to let the baby out.

Tearing is natural and heals better *providing* it does not go too far (although many still dispute this). Episiotomy induces a sense of assault, however well intentioned, on an area very private to you. This feeling of assault can spread to the whole body. The homoeopathic remedy that often heals this trauma is Staphisagria. A few doses will release the anger and the abused feeling, and save the woman from feeling violated, especially when sexual relations restart. (After a hysterectomy many women never have sex again and the feeling of assault or loss is probably a strong reason for this, as it is likely to resurface again during attempts to make love.) As many people are very ill at ease when expressing or articulating their feelings, especially about such sensitive matters, once caused they may never be resolved without help.

A Caesarean can often leave a mother in deep anger. If this is not expressed it can go inside as depression and become the familiar postpartum syndrome.

A delivery that is slow to start may reflect a reluctance on the part of the mother to let go. Deepseated separation traumas might be surfacing here and Pulsatilla could help.

Arnica deals very effectively with physical trauma and the emotions surrounding it. It is therefore useful during birth for the pain of contractions, which it softens, and can be a great help afterwards.

BIRTH AND INFANCY

Separation at birth and afterwards

Separation can occur at birth. The baby is put in the nursery for a few days; they are fed by the nurses but left alone, with no one to be close to. Some babies experience several days of separation at birth when the mother needs to sleep and recover from a 'bad' birth. It is not uncommon either for unwell babies to spend up to a month in an incubator, only seeing their mother infrequently during this period.

In my experience isolation in an incubator is often an extremely damaging experience psychologically and leaves the baby wounded for life, feeling fundamentally and deeply alone (see Stramonium pattern in Chapter 9 and isolation in the indexes in Chapter 8). My conclusion is that incubators should not be used. There is a better way. In one country they ran out of incubators so they got the mothers to tie the premature babies to their bodies. To the doctors' surprise these babies survived better than those in the incubators.

Because the deep nature of these traumas is not appreciated, however, the child receives attention but never enough to recover, as the parents do not understand the extent of the damage that has been done. So there is a double bind in the isolation experience and no means of recovery from it. The crisis becomes a catastrophe. Knowing this can help if you are a new mother or father of a premature baby. Such children need endless physical and emotional contact, a sling not a cot, to sleep with you, not separated from you, as described in the book *The Continuum Concept* (essential reading for parents).

Such separations can result in people who as adults are seriously depressive, suicidal perhaps, or very anxious about everything, anorexic, panicky, ill, criminally inclined or deeply religious. Society may imprison them or they may imprison themselves, for example in the church or in a disease, but few will relate the later posture, attitude or disease to the birth separation.

Absent fathers can also cause traumas. The father often leaves the family with feelings of betrayal, loss, grief, rejection and more. He may go to war, or die from sickness or from an accident. More often he will leave because the marriage is not working or because he has fallen in love with someone else. Even when the father is around physically, he is often not there for the child because of work commitments, etc. Even when he is there and available, the father's role in our society is so obscure that few know what to do with their children.

For any of these reasons and many others, fathers and mothers are 'absent' or leave their children. The children may be extremely upset, without the parents realizing it, and become severely traumatized. If parents really appreciated the pain that children can suffer from their separations, and the traumas inflicted, there might be fewer break-ups. But staying together in guilt solves nothing; it just adds another bind.

Adoption

Adoption is a very difficult process to emerge from un-traumatized. Take this example.

A girl falls in love with a foreign visitor and becomes pregnant. Initially all is well and they plan to marry. Then a letter arrives from the boyfriend's wife. Shock, rage, betrayal, deep disappointment and deep distress result. Her parents want her to have the baby adopted. At three weeks old the baby is handed over, but the mother continues to visit. For a year the 'birth mother' remains undecided as to whether to let the child go or not. The adopting parents inevitably hold back, as they cannot let all their love flow with all the uncertainty. Finally the decision is made.

Thirty years on the grown man has had a string of broken relationships and has suffered great disappointments in love. He is now in a push–pull situation between a new lover and his regular girlfriend, unable to make up his mind. This situation mirrors his feelings from the adoption, the struggle. Likewise, the repeated disappointments reflect the mother's trauma when he was in the womb.

A baby boy was rejected at birth and put in an orphanage where he was kept permanently in a cot – fed and watered and cleaned but nothing else – *for a whole year*. Then a woman adopted him, an older, professional single woman who wanted a child to bring up. She was told there was nothing wrong with him. It turned out that he had terrible tinnitus, noises in his ears that drove him to distraction. By eight years old he could not hear. He had never spoken a word but was continually in pain, grimacing, holding his ears in a permanent state of suffering, day and night.

He would pull at his clothes or cling desperately to his adopted mother, never wanting her to leave him, full of fear, waking frequently at night screaming, and with a great fear of the dark. The EEG was normal and no specialist knew what to do.

Stramonium was obviously indicated. It was given as directed in this book and in two days he calmed down, slept all night, heard his first word and said 'Mummy' for the first time in his life.

Reflecting parental troubles

Although nine months in the womb can be a trauma, if there is a generally loving environment during the pregnancy and things go well, including the birth, then the child can come out basically feeling well. However, if the parents then start to react with their own traumatized responses or tension arises between them, the child can start to reflect these problems. They can react to any feeling they experience as hurtful with anger and fear and grief expressed as crying, whining and waking often. If these traumas are strong they can develop symptoms and diseases which reflect the parental feeling rather than their own problems.

In this situation it is really up to the parent to put their own intuition to work at the infant's level and to understand what the infant is complaining about through their very limited repertoire of expression.

When children are older and logic, talking and reason come into play there is a shift towards increasing self-responsibility, but initially it is up to the parent to sort out their own problems and to stop inflicting them on their children.

Colic

Colic is a common complaint of infants and is frequently due to suppressed rage. The child may be picking up on unexpressed anger. Perhaps the mother needs Staphisagria for an episiotomy or other birth traumas or Sepia for stifled affections. Alternatively the child may need Colocynthus, which is the main homoeopathic remedy for doubling up, twisting, griping, intensely agonizing colic and, like Staphisagria is useful for suppressed anger traumas and their effects.

Loss of Sleep

In the mother or father, loss of sleep for a long period, owing to a frequently waking baby, can become a temporary trauma, and if sleep time cannot be found, it eventually becomes a permanent problem. A year of lost sleep can be devastating. Cocculus can help resolve this, although obviously practical measures are also necessary.

Weakness

Weakness from loss of blood or diarrhoea or other body fluids can often be remedied by China, the main homoeopathic remedy for physical exhaustion from loss of body fluids.

A woman was very weak after childbirth, with an ulcer about two inches across spreading out on her leg. Homoeopathic remedies were used, but to no avail. Then in a dream, she met a homoeopath who suggested she take China; she did and it cured the ulcer in about a day. So if you have well-developed inner connections to higher aspects of yourself or to nature and you receive information from these sources, they might reveal your essential life drama, your core trauma or the remedy needed. My patients give me such symbolic information to guide or determine the remedy choice.

Jealousy

A first child is often not wanted, or is the wrong sex, or was the reason the parents married, and can be blamed for the problem.

If a second child then comes, who is of the right sex, or planned and wanted, or if one parent bonds strongly with the second then the first child will often experience intense jealousy, needing the homoeopathic remedy Lachesis. A grown man with jealous children may exhibit classic Lachesis symptoms, being slightly dishevelled, extremely talkative and admitting a strong irrational fear of snakes. This could be his infant trauma of jealousy showing itself in himself and his children.

TRAUMA IN ADULTHOOD

Panic attacks

A forty-year-old computer salesman came to see me with skin complaints, broken red veins on his face and blocked sinuses.

After some treatments that seemed to be ineffective, he related this story to me, which had been told to him by his aunt. When he was six weeks old his mother left him in the bath briefly to answer the phone and he turned over. He very nearly drowned.

He also told me of recurring dreams of choking, which he had clearly not related to the near-drowning. He also often talked of drowning in paperwork at work and the blocked sinuses seemed on reflection to be the main problem.

Faced with situations like this I often imagine myself in the trauma position. You might like to try this. Imagine that your hands are behind your back as you lie face down in a bath and you are helpless to keep your head out of the water. You breathe in; but all you get is water. You are choking. In this way you can gain an insight into the experience of it.

Given a very caring parent, this might have been mended, but clearly his dreams, the words he used and the blocked sinuses indicated that it was not. It seemed to me all related.

Terror after being left in the dark

A girl of four years slept in the summerhouse on summer evenings. The parents would be out in the garden and the mother would go over and check that she was all right every ten minutes or so. As darkness fell, she would put a light on as the child was afraid of the dark.

One evening, being busy with something the mother forgot to check for some time. It had become dark by this time and the girl was awake and screaming. The mother said she knew instantly that something had happened in her child, something important, something she, the mother, could not identify, but clearly the child was deeply affected. For a long time the child woke in the night with nightmares and then they subsided.

Many years later when she was ten or so, she came to see me with nightmares again. There had been another event in the child's life. The parents had separated and the same problem had resurfaced. If the traumas are similar enough the old ones are reactivated. Here they were both traumatic separations.

Her dream, now she was old enough to relate it, included black objects and waking in terror which, put together with her intense dislike of being alone after dark, indicated Stramonium, which was given with complete success. Not only did the terrorizing dreams go, but she was able to go camping, which is similar to being out in the summerhouse, something she had always previously refused to do. Many subtle changes like this showed how deeply the wound had been healed.

Stramonium is a very common remedy for children with night terrors. My guess is that the original trauma here was to do with birth.

The terror of inner violence

A man came to see me with stomach troubles. His expression was cheerful and smiling, and he was joking. He was a single man, having left his wife and daughter.

He seemed on the defensive and I felt intuitively that he was violent inside. After some time building up trust, I enquired about any fantasies he might have. Eventually he admitted that he had violent fantasies. I then dropped the subject, as I could see I was pushing him too hard, and pursued less contentious subjects, returning later via another route to his anger.

I asked him about his separation and visits to his daughter. He admitted that he did not see his daughter much. When I enquired why, he evaded the question, but much later in the interview he suddenly volunteered that he did not live with her any more as he was scared of hitting her and that this was the first time he had realized this. I guessed that his father had been violent, hitting him as a child, and he confirmed this. I realized that his cheerful, smiling posture was a ploy to deflect violence: 'look at me, I am happy and smiling so there is no reason to hit me', an intelligent defensive posture as a child.

Here then was a father for whom the 'mirror' of his child was too much to bear. He left to avoid hitting her. The child meanwhile probably feels rejected and grows up missing her father. What sort of men will she choose, I wonder? With this rejection and the father's latent violence, I would guess that she would choose violent men who would beat her and then reject her. This situation is typical of the remedy Nux vomica.

Serious assault

Muggings and sudden assaults by persons unknown can cause terror and the homoeopathic remedy Stramonium is frequently the answer. Here is one such story.

A young woman student was attacked and raped and the attacker then decided to strangle her to avoid being identified. She lost consciousness but he panicked and ran off. Afterwards she could not sleep at all without the light full on and a friend in the room. She was full of terror, totally overwhelmed. There may have been rage and fury underneath but the first stage was terror, stark terror as she was expecting to be murdered on losing consciousness.

Stramonium acted immediately and she could sleep normally. In the next phase of recovery Staphisagria was needed for the rage as and when it surfaced after the terror dissolved.

Held at gunpoint

A man was attacked and held alone at gunpoint in a isolated farmhouse. The attacker told him it was execution time. He loaded two bullets into the gun and pointed it at his head, as he lay tied up on the floor. The attacker pulled the trigger. Nothing happened. The attacker was playing games; he had put the bullets in and secretly removed them again.

The man was terrified. He was a poet and had a stutter that was strongest on the first words, both classic indications for the homoeopathic remedy Stramonium. I concluded that this was a replay event reflecting previous traumas in his life. Stramonium was extremely effective so somewhere inside was a very deeply wounded child, terrorized by something I did not need to find out about then. I find it hard to believe that this was an 'action replay' of an actual event and not just a coincidence as logic would suggest. Yet Stramonium had been his remedy for most if not all his life; the facts were clear, and this terrorizing incident clearly needed Stramonium too.

My experience of 'action replays' confounds this more universal interpretation of coincidence, because 'action replays' take place so often and fit so well with what goes on in so many lives.

Shock in war

This is the story of a United Nations soldier in 1993.

His brigade was sent as peace keepers into a war zone. At one point he was in the trenches for seventeen days without sleep; as he put it, 'It was too dangerous to sleep.' He was selected as one of a crew to reconnoitre in an armoured vehicle, but at the last minute he was told he was not going and someone else took his place. The armoured vehicle suffered a direct hit and one soldier, his friend, was literally blown to pieces. Another solider was injured and the rest crawled out. The subject of this tale was given the job of retrieving the dead and wounded. He had to pick up the dismembered pieces of his friend and bring them out.

After this experience he was in severe shock. He was sent home after some time on drugs and his wife said he did not know where he was or who she was. He was in a severely disorientated state. He suffered headaches and stomach pains every day since then, and four months after the event, he could sleep only briefly with hypnotic drugs, but better with alcohol, which provided two hours' sleep.

He is a stocky, strong man with great fear in his eyes. His wife told me that he had been like this since he arrived home, and she was also suffering. He was afraid to be alone at all. He was afraid something would happen. He had a great fear accompanied by heart palpitations. When questioned as to what he feared precisely he replied that he was especially afraid that his heart would stop and that it could happen any time; any minute he would die. He was also constantly thinking, 'It could have been me in that armoured vehicle, how was it I was spared?'

Before this event he had always been healthy. I discovered, however, that he was born a twin two months premature.

The doctors did not realize there was another baby, and the twin therefore came out too late and soon died. So his first experience of life was the death of the person then closest to him, and but for fate it could have been him. I now realized why this war trauma had struck in so deeply. It had re-awakened his earliest life trauma. His first life experience was sudden death and the 'it could have been me' idea. It was a deep forgotten memory. To cap that initial trauma, he then spent thirty days in isolation in an incubator. Only then could he received good loving parenting.

That was his story. The analysis was easy once everything was understood.

Shock
Death expected at any minute.
Fear of death during palpitations.
Alcohol relaxes the fear.

Aconite was the remedy. He took it the same evening and slept until ten o'clock next morning, something which was previously impossible. His pains stopped and he continued to improve. The power of homoeopathic remedies is totally amazing when you witness it in such situations.

Interestingly, his neighbour's wife sat in on the consultation, which was actually an evening meal, and she said afterwards that her husband had also been in the army. He was now retired, but he had had a similar experience, and he had not slept properly in twenty years.

Betrayal and secrets

Betrayal – being let down by a close friend, parent or partner, and similar slights – can sometimes go very deep and highlight primitive traumas that occurred long ago. Here is such a case.

A detective came to see me with irritable bowel syndrome. After hearing his story, it became clear that his main life issue was that, at the age of twelve, on Christmas Day, he was told that he was adopted. That was all he was told. Nothing else was said. What a day to drop a bombshell like that and then pretend that everything was fine. But he was very angry at being so deceived, and the trauma was deduced to be 'betrayal causing grief and humiliation'.

That he was informed so inappropriately, without preparation or discussion, was, it seemed to me, the cornerstone of the case, especially when I took into account his job – a detective, one who seeks out deception or betrayal. There were also other clear pieces of confirmatory information.

Putting betrayal, humiliation, a passion for work and a few other signs together made this a clear Nux vomica case. That was the nature of the wound. Nux vomica can be cruel, hard, and unfeeling, in just the way the wound was inflicted. This is also how the victim of such behaviour can become. Nux vomica is made from a nut rich in strychnine, itself a spasmodic drug, inducing spasmodic behaviour quite similar to the peculiarities of his symptoms – 'irritable bowel syndrome'.

Keeping the identity of the parent secret

There are deeper betrayal issues too, to do with deception and conception. It is current practice, when the man is infertile, to use artificial insemination from sperm that cannot be traced and to recommend that the child never be told; to leave the child to assume that the 'father' is the real father. I and others feel that this is very wrong, burdening the person for life with a disconnection, a lie.

I feel that all fathers and mothers should be traceable. The mother has the child inside her for the first nine months of its life and that is a vitally important time, and an important basis for its own process. A father can still have a profound influence in my experience, even when he does not know that he conceived a child.

As an example, an adopted woman only met her real mother once, and later went to her funeral. Around the grave stood a group of relatives she had never met before, yet who moved, spoke, and looked just like herself, in stark contrast to her adopted family. It gave her a deep sense of belonging, a deep connective feeling.

I feel strongly that it is best not to have secrets. They

always seem to create an emotional distance, keeping you on your guard. It is always a potential problem, leading perhaps to a deep wound some time in the future. And I think that somewhere, deep inside, the deceived person always knows it. Discussion can be a point of strength, growth and trust.

Relationship break-up

A partner can feel betrayed when a relationship breaks up. They can feel that the other partner has broken all the previously agreed commitments, the unwritten trust and just gone off and done their own thing regardless.

They may go over and over the events in their thoughts, unable to get them out of their mind (classic Nat mur). The greatest difficulty is often that their ex-partner would have been the very one to whom they were closest to and to whom they would normally talk about such things.

They may start to hate the other person, and this may develop into feelings of hurting or killing, stabbing with a knife, or conversely loss of feeling. They may feel very angry inside but be unable to express the anger in any external way. In these circumstances it frequently shows as churning thoughts, aggressive feelings or actions, or possibly swearing. These processes are very common in divorce and other situation where great trust is shattered.

Pretending a crisis has not happened

Parents frequently betray their children by pretending that a crisis has not happened. Children are not allowed to see a dead parent or relative or go to the funeral, or are told nothing about the death. I have heard many stories of pretended that death has not happened. The child is sent away to a relative for the duration of the grieving process and the dead person is never talked about afterwards. The father may have committed suicide and the child is never told. He lives permanently with the feeling that something terrible is going to happen, yet with no tangible reason for it. How are these deceived children able to say goodbye, to grieve, to make sense of it all, to rearrange their lives?

Violence

An eight-year-old boy who comes to see me is capable of extreme violence. He seems to attract it. He walks into a playground and other children, strangers to him, attack him.

At home he can beat down doors and terrify his single-parent mother. He likewise terrorizes teachers, social workers, workers in childrens' homes and educational advisers, for when he lets rip there is trouble. No one can contain him in his rages, when his strength is greatly increased.

When I have been with this child he sometimes looks at me with a hard stare, eyeing me up with a streak of cold detachment, a hint of real cruelty. He doodles wolves with sharp teeth.

His mother has a pathological lack of confidence. She originally came to see me for sinusitis, the after-effects of a broken nose from being beaten up.

The father was serving life imprisonment for deliberate cold-blooded murder. He was caught red-handed, having stabbed a stranger forty times or so and yet he never admitted it.

The trauma this boy suffered seemed to be inherited from both sides. On one side we have the mother, with pathological inferiority based on violence experienced as a child; on the other, the murderous father and also the near certainty that he had pathological inferiority with a murderous reflex based on experiencing extreme violence as a child. Both these fit the homoeopathic remedy picture of Anacardium. Murderous rage, extreme cruelty, an evil intent and serious lack of confidence are its hallmarks.

I would imagine that this child found getting love from his mother difficult because of her own extremely wounded state. In fact, he must have felt that only violence really made him feel alive, noticed, visible, human. I would think his experiences at conception and in the womb left him little option but to feel separated and alone in the world, isolated from everyone, as if no one else existed, for this is the underlying feeling of the Anacardium picture.

As far as I could see, and his mother confirmed this, Anacardium outperformed the hospital specialists, the child psychologists, the teachers, the social workers and the special care units.

Sexual abuse

This term can be used for widely different situations but I use it to cover all situations where an adult has inappropriate sexual contact with a child. There are, however, three over-lapping but distinct areas: sexual contact with an infant who is too young to remember, which is the most difficult to recover from; sexual contact which is blotted out initially but can be clearly remembered once it is safe to do so; and sexual contact which usually involves a teenager and which is never forgotten but needs a safe place to resolve the trauma.

The situation varies according to whether the abuser is a stranger, a close relative or a family friend. Sexual abuse usually takes place within the home and is frequently per-petrated by the parents, close relatives, boyfriends, close family friends and child carers such as babysitters. Women violate their sons sexually, as do men their daughters and sons. Both are much more common than we appreciate.

Often both parents are involved; one does it and the other turns a blind eye or is also a victim of abuse. Abusers are likely to have been abused in the past. Violent people and abusers share many characteristics.

Denial

If someone is sexually abused by their father at a very young age, they may hate him for it but also still love him, two perfectly valid yet contradictory feelings. If he says it is a special secret, just between the two of them then it can be too much for the chld to contain in their conscious mind. Often the only recourse is to deny that anything happened. They may remember in later life or, if not, start acting it out on others.

Denial can take another form with parents. If the child tries to talk to the other parent they may stick up for their spouse and even beat the child for 'telling lies'.

Denial that abuse is happening or has happened is appropriate until the person can get to a place where they feel safe enough to deal with it. This may take an hour, a month, a year or twenty years. The emotions that cause the memory to stay locked away and denied involve the conflict between being hurt yourself and hurting the perpetrator and possibly destroying the whole family fabric. The family can end up living a lie, perhaps with the father and daughter unable to talk because of the ever-present threat of their secret being revealed.

Self-blame

The victim may believe that they are somehow to blame themselves, that they encouraged the abuse or invited it, especially if they initially enjoyed it or the special relationship with their father.

Acting out the abuse

Self-hate can manifest as drug abuse, suicidal tendencies, self-mutilation, rage and the desire to kill someone close. There could also be panic attacks.

'Action replays' of this abuse trauma can resurface in a mother when her girl reaches the age at which she was abused. The mother might then become overwhelmingly emotional as she recovers some of the repressed feelings, without yet knowing where they come from.

Denied feelings can promote numbness, or there can be excessive sexual behaviour arising out of the confusion between sexuality and the safety of the child–parent relationship. Likewise, there can be numerous sexual fixations. The secret can remain very deep, resulting in all sorts of fears and fantasy states and mental delusions. There may be deep resentments and an aversion to men or women. Aversion to or estrangement from family, whether the whole family or only some members, is common.

The experience of abuse spreads like a web throughout the abused person and the whole family, contaminating them on many levels of existence.

Disease as a result

After abuse the victim will often try to cut the experience out of their mind, out of sight. This denial effectively withdraws energy from the abused area by paying no attention to it. This can weaken the area and restrict its normal recovery from infection. For example, we now know that directing warm positive feelings repeatedly to an affected area helps healing. Conversely, then, the permanent unconscious revulsion of one particular area of the body can cause the opposite.

Because the genital area is where the abuse was centred the denial may result in feelings being cut off from there or stored up there and many problems are likely in this region. Any type of female problem, such as period pain, sexual difficulties, infertility, vaginismus, cystitis, thrush or PMT, endometriosis, which persists for a long time, may indicate abuse. Sexual problems in men, such as failure of erections or low sex urge, could also have their origin in abuse. Some sexual abuse is anal, so any anal symptoms may result from it too.

PARENTAL INFLUENCES UPON TRAUMA

There is a very large group of traumas which are not caused by a sudden event but by a slow insidious process to which the person has no answer.

Put-downs

These arise from the parent telling the child he or she is 'no good' in some way. Initially the child will stand up to these but if the parent reinforces the message with treats or punishment, the child gives up. They lose faith in themselves and in the world in general to some extent.

Continuous put-downs can have a lasting effect on self-confidence and repeatedly devaluing a child can bring about distress which, if not counterbalanced, can bring trauma.

Specific approval

Another classic trauma occurs when a child learns early on that love is only really given for achievements. The trauma could result in the child always seeking approval for their inventive, unusual or strange behaviour, or for their specialist knowledge.

One type of trauma caused by this conditioning is treated by the homoeopathic remedy Lycopodium. These people may learn that appreciation and love come through intellectual pursuits. Doing well at school gets them credit and approval so learning becomes the route to love. Here thinking is valued over feelings, as was graphically illustrated in the film *Dead Poets Society*.

No cuddles, no confidence

Behind every childhood trauma there must surely lie a lack of affection, contact, quality attention and manifest loving, as Jean Liedloff in *The Continuum Concept* so vividly depicts.

Many traumas arise from having parents who feed and clothe their child but who are not present emotionally. The children are brushed off with nannies, nurseries and boarding schools resulting in anger, grief and rejection. The child feels that the world is unsafe and lonely and grows up feeling deeply insecure in intangible ways.

I believe that lack of loving is the most common childhood experience in the west.

Mirroring

When your child plays your own traumas back to you, it can be a great teaching mirror for you. They can show you every fixation you ever had. They can almost force you to look at the secret hidden issues you would normally ignore. They can be the actors of your 'action replays' and they can continue to be so throughout their lives, unless you attend to your traumas. They are a tremendously rich experience which you cannot escape from, unless you suppress your child, as is common. I cited elsewhere typical examples of parents who could not take the mirroring.

Given emotional support, quality listening, interaction, appreciation and love, your child will allow you to revisit and re-experience your own history and to rework it and make yourself anew into a more conscious being. They are sometimes better, more accurate and more direct than any healer or therapist, and are always there for you and free!

Visits to grandparents can also be quite revealing for the parents. Your parents often start treating the grandchild as they treated you, especially if the grandchild is the same sex, and you can observe firsthand how you were treated.

Typical childhood scripts

A script is a typical form of behaviour taken up as a way of survival in childhood. It can condition you for life. For example the firstborn child often takes after the mother, the second after the father. This is more pronounced when parents fit gender stereotypes and when it is girl first and boy second. When the parents are more equal and less polarized, working together in harmony, this effect is reduced and all the children will tend to draw from both parents as role models.

If the father is absent, the first child can start feeling that they should fill his role even as early as five. The first boy, as an adult, might feel that he is head of the family and act that role when in reality he might be the most traumatized of all the children.

TRAUMAS FROM DYSFUNCTIONAL PARENTING

A two-year-old who grabs a toy from another child does not think of the pain of rejection or frustration of purpose the other child will be feeling. He thinks of the loss he feels when he sees his favourite toy in another's hands. He does not yet have the recall that will tell him that there is a strong probability that the toy will be restored to him shortly (that knowledge is born of experience and the increasing ability to recollect). He is totally in the moment and will most probably protest strongly.

Until someone has built up an understanding of their own feelings and how these can effectively be dealt with, they are unable to consider the feelings of others. They literally do not have the ability. The toddler snatching a toy without malice but with a clear conviction of his own feelings will be quite open to any new experience such as his parent offering him something even better in exchange for the toy. If this kind of uncritical response happens often enough he will gradually become more open to alternative ways of responding to that type of situation.

On the other hand, any whiff of criticism (and children are highly sensitive and finely tuned to criticism, experiences being new to them and taken at face value) will create in them a feeling of discomfort. Our first reaction to discomfort is to close up a little in defence, thus creating a preoccupation with ourselves (dealing with the problem of the immediate discomfort). This leaves less room in our consciousness for consideration of the other person. Well-meaning attempts to encourage consideration for others in a child who has not yet reached that stage of development are therefore counterproductive.

A loving parent who shows their love but at the same time shows disappointment in the child's behaviour (often a deep disappointment) will be giving their child the message that they love them in spite of the fact that they are not good enough. The child will therefore accept without question that they are not good enough; after all, they have it on the best authority, that of the person who loves them best in the whole world. The toddler whose parent thinks he was behaving 'badly' cannot therefore correctly interpret the adult's concern; he cannot understand the complicated mixture of responses raised in the adult by seeing their child behave antisocially. He has not yet reached a level of comprehension to grasp it all.

Similarly, a seven-year-old who is shouted at by his mother as they leave for school for forgetting something he needs may well not yet have reached the level of maturity necessary to take responsibility for such things. He just receives the message that he was not good enough, that he has failed.

We all do this in some way or another because we are all human and under pressure. We are, however, adults with an adult's comprehension, and if we understand that the results of what we do are not the results that we are looking for, then we are in a better position to correct the situation.

Some stories of parental trauma

When I was visiting a friend one day we sat down to lunch, four adults and their seven-year-old daughter. The daughter was was the only child of proud parents and was born when they were well into their thirties. Before the meal had progressed far the child, who was delicate and fine and usually not at all clumsy, accidentally knocked over her water. Both parents' voices were immediately raised in censure: 'Geraldine, you clumsy girl, how careless, go and get a cloth at once!' came loudly from the father, and 'Oh, Geraldine! You silly girl,' with sorrow from her mother. As an adult I reeled under the impact and intensity of their response and I had not even done it! The full effect on a sensitive and aware child who had made a small mistake is hard to guess.

Her immediate response would have been to recoil under the blow, to draw herself in physically by tightening her muscles, as if in protection. We all do this as a natural instinctive response to attack, whether physical or verbal. The result of this tensing is to constrict the lungs. Our breathing is therefore reduced so that the oxygen supply to our bodies is limited and this causes reduced efficiency in the whole body system.

Why did those parents react like this? I am sure that all three, including the child, regarded it as a minor everyday mishap giving rise to inconvenience and therefore irritation for the parents, and perhaps some embarrassment in front of visitors. What I do not think they were aware of was the severity of the reaction in relation to the seriousness of what had happened. Why did it matter so much? All three were also probably unaware of the child's physical reaction.

The significance of this kind of incident in health terms is the way the body deals with the effects of it. As the day wore on it is probable that if this were an isolated incident the child would gradually forget how uncomfortable she had felt and the whole thing would be wiped from her mind until she found herself in a similar situation, perhaps the next time her parents shouted at her. It is here that the significance of relatively minor trauma lies. Two things could have happened. Either Geraldine's discomfort could gradually have faded and receded; later in the day when her parents were relaxed, one of them might have spent some quality time with her, doing something together or reading to her and having a cuddle, for instance, where she would have experienced both physically and emotionally her parents' acceptance and love for her. The remnants of her muscular tensing would have relaxed with this and her body would be restored to well-being and to its full functioning.

Imagine, however, that as the day wore on the parents became increasingly tense themselves. It is quite easy to visualize that under these circumstances the next small mistake the little girl made would call forth a similar response to the first. This time it would have a slightly greater effect as she would already be tense, hurting and uncomfortable from the first telling-off.

I knew a fourteen-year-old girl from a middle-class family, with one parent a teacher and the other an intellectual, who even at her age had trouble and experienced distress trying to fathom which of her natural responses were acceptable to the adults around her (whether at school, at home or in other people's homes). From babyhood she had sometimes experienced great affection and show of love: rewards for doing well, presents when her mother was feeling good and wanted to indulge her. She had also experienced rejection when behaviour appropriate to her age was inconvenient for her mother. In a voluble and passionate family this rejection was as chilling and as deep as the show of love was warm and comfortable. Neither was a predictable or comprehensible response appropriate to her behaviour but rather a reflection of her parents' moods. So she found herself sometimes indulged, sometimes heavily criticized but she could never accurately predict which would come and this left her in a permanent state of apprehension and therefore tension.

This is a common state in children whose parents' responses to their children are determined by their own emotional state at the time more than by the children's behaviour. This is baffling to the children, who find that sometimes 'No' means 'No and you'll get a clip around the ears if you don't take notice'; sometimes it means 'Not at the moment but if you go on pestering long enough you'll get what you want because I haven't the strength to deal with you'; and sometimes it means nothing more than 'I don't want to see you doing it but as long as I am not put to any trouble it doesn't matter what you do'.

The products of such upbringings are seriously confused and anxious people, unsure whether their behaviour is going to bring reward or censure. These children will either be confused and angry, rebelling against their parents and any form of authority (this is the core of many of the problems in schools today), or they will be overanxious through their inability to learn from experience what makes them acceptable and will have become uncharacteristically timid and fearful of trying new things.

Three-and-a-half-year-old Henry came to visit us one day with his mother (a health visitor with two children and a comfortable home and a good marriage). He went with my children into the garden and we followed with our cups of coffee. In the garden we had a fairly large pond less than half a metre deep, with a gravel beach at both ends and a bridge over the middle.

Henry ran happily along the path with the other children, who went onto the bridge. As his mother saw where they were going she stiffened beside me and called out anxiously, 'Be careful Henry' and made as if to rush after him. I assured her that the pond was shallow (and we were ourselves only a few feet away) and she turned nervously to me and told me how worried she was about the children hurting themselves. Still watching tensely, she told me how her other child was clumsy and accident-prone.

I observed Henry's face cloud over and lose its look of spontaneous joy when he first heard the anxiety in his mother's call and saw how cautiously he had trod up the two little steps in the path before coming to the bridge whereas he had only moments before skipped up a run of about five steps as freely and agilely as the other children. The mother was conveying her excessive anxiety to her child, inhibiting his natural ability to use his body free from tension and to learn by his experience so that he was being forced to some extent to live his life through her.

I have deliberately chosen this minor everyday incident, which would perhaps not be termed trauma, to illustrate just how easily quite serious tension can build up in a child. Needless to say, such stresses accumulate in the same way in an adult with the pressures of adult responsibility and modern living. When you picture these incidents occurring daily, often frequently throughout the day, you begin to see the permanent disadvantage under which the body is labouring.

A girl who at the age of two had watched her mother being beaten almost to death had not started to speak properly when she started school. Until seven or eight years old she was classed as having speech problems. I saw her at the age of nine and was told that she had never received any form of help for her psychological problems because she was just one amongst so many and on the whole her behaviour had settled down as her speech improved and she was not as much trouble as some of the other children.

This child is carrying the horror of seeing her mother beaten through her life without any recognition of her pain, with no one ever having acknowledged that what she felt and still feels regarding it are normal reactions, not her private, desperate secret and strange peculiarity. Yet she had clearly indicated her distress for years and years: a tiny child who has felt the unspeakable helplessness of being the only witness to extreme violence visited upon the mother she loves and utterly helpless at the age of two to do anything to prevent it, showing that helpless frustration in her total inability to speak for years. Was her later gradual development of language due to a slow building up of trust in something or someone?

I think the above examples show that apparently normal parenting but with violence or confusion over parental messages of approval and disapproval a backdrop can result in fear. And fear is the most damaging of feelings to live with; it is the basis of psychological damage that cannot be overestimated, resulting in loss of confidence and loss of interest, often lasting a lifetime.

SCHOOLS

John Taylor Gatto, New York Teacher of the Year 1991, said this in his acceptance speech:

> Although teachers do care and do work hard, very hard, the institution is psychopathic; it has no conscience, and if the bell rings when a young man is in the middle of writing a poem he must stop and move to a different cell ... We must realize that school does 'schooling' very well ... Children learn to obey orders but it does not educate. This possibility is pre-empted by the design of schools ... Children lose virtually every sign of curiosity.

Boarding school

Boarding school is often a long-drawn-out trauma resulting in the cutting off of feelings.

A child was brought to me from a very prominent boarding school. He was suffering from lack of access to his parents, plus abuse at school. In the first term the school deliberately sought to restrict access to the parents so as to settle the child in. This was the script, breaking the tie of feeling and support, teaching the pupil to discount feelings and 'be a man'. His illness stemmed from this.

When I pointed out that the child was suffering from being at this school, the father basically said, in true public school fashion, 'I went there. I hated it, but it was good for me, so it is good for him.' In other words, he had been programmed not to respect his feelings or anybody else's.

Another sufferer, a senior official in local government with permanent physical injuries resulting from indiscriminate use of the cane, described boarding school as a brutalizing experience.

DISEASE IMPRINT TRAUMA

It is common knowledge in homoeopathy that diseases of past generations can affect current and future ones. I call it disease imprint trauma and I believe it to be a distortion of or damage to the psychological and physical immune system. Medical science is beginning to think that all chronic diseases are slow viruses. Diabetes, for example, is a lifelong process that only becomes apparent when it is far advanced or when trauma damage weakens the immune system. Homoeopathy often has an effective answer to these processes.

The most common diseases with dramatic after-effects are tuberculosis, cancer and gonorrhoea (including non-specific urethritis (NSU) which is gonorrhoea muted by antibiotics). Samuel Hahnemann added two more: syphilis and what he called psora, which is really suppressed vitality causd by a number of things, including drugs used to suppress skin complaints. In such situations the person's energy drops and they permanently underfunction. Psora is really a catch-all concept for all the multifarious reasons why people underfunction.

Tuberculosis (TB) leaves damage which encourages relapsing conditions such as what is now called ME, a generalized malaise that is not clearly definable. (ME is also similar to a non-paralytic form of polio and may only have occurred since the advent of polio vaccination, which might yet prove to be a causative factor.)

Tubercular types have simple pictures which are well drawn in the trauma pattern section. For example when there is a disease imprint of TB, the subject may travel the world several times. Travelling is a strong pointer to a tubercular disease imprint. All the children may do it or just one, which shows that the disease imprint is not always activated. In one such person there may be recurring dreams of escaping on long train journeys to other countries or in children a tendency to run off in the supermarket at any opportunity, in stark contrast to those children with separation issues, who will cling on and never let the parent out of their sight.

Children and adults with the tubercular disease imprint type are often scared of dogs and grind their teeth at night, and the infants have terrible tantrums. They frequently develop colds and acute illnesses and fail to thrive if the tubercular disease imprint is not dealt with.

Tubercular types are also more prone to cancer and it is therefore desirable to reduce or eliminate the tubercular profile early in life if possible. It seems that the tubercular disease imprint, which is some sort of immune system malfunction, allows cancer to develop more readily or provides the psychological conditions for it. For example, tubercular types are very stubborn and this might bring about long-held and deep resentments, which are one cause of cancer. Frequently a woman holding a grudge against her partner will get a lump in her breast.

Gonorrhoea is indicated in emotionally driven people who generally do things to excess. They tend to overindulge in everything from drugs to sex to parties. They feel most comfortable sleeping on their fronts, tend to love the sea and animals, and as infants have fiery red nappy rashes (see Medorrhinum).

Cancer types by contrast can be unemotional and unexpressive and do not develop the usual childhood diseases; instead they often have other severe illness such as several bad doses of pneumonia. They too like the sea and animals and prefer to sleep on their fronts. Cancer types have a very wide range of symptoms but they have a unique picture which is easily recognizable by a homoeopath and is detailed in the section on trauma pictures. Often there will be a strong history of cancer in the family. Cancer may sit on top of a previous gonorrhoea history which may sit on top of a tubercular history, each one laying the foundations for the next.

Syphilitic types are self-destructive, going in for any number of activities that destroy them, such as alcoholism.

Disease imprints do not mean that the person will automatically get the disease. However, they will be more prone to it; for example, a gonorrhoea type may more easily contract the disease if infected, and they will run more risk of getting the infection through their excessive behaviour. They will also find it more difficult to cure the infection than a person without the disease imprint.

There is little doubt in my mind that most therapeutic processes have no real answers to these inherited disease traumas, especially if they are strong, and the appropriate homoeopathic disease imprint remedy is frequently needed to erase the trauma, otherwise it will continue to fester.

POISONING TRAUMAS

Any metal can create a poisoning picture in a person but this can often be substantially alleviated if the pathology is not already too far advanced, sometimes by giving the poison in homoeopathic potency. Alzheimer's disease may be associated with aluminium, which gets into the body from cooking pots and fast food containers, and is almost unavoidable when eating out. Mercury comes from dental fillings, lead from old printing presses, silver from developing black and white photographs with unprotected hands. All can be treated. Silver poisoning can be avoided by using thin disposable gloves. Dental fillings may need complete replacement with plastic ones in sensitive people. Typically, people with mercury poisoning can have a mouth full of ulcers, which resist cure with any treatment until the fillings are all removed.

DRUG TRAUMA

The following is a real case history, as it occurred.

The patient's verrucas had been burned off using medication prescribed by a doctor. After two years, the subject had glandular fever and could not work for a while. There were also arthritic pains in the fingers. After another two years, large red blotches appeared on the skin and were suppressed with steroids.

Then the subject developed ulcerative colitis and ME. The drug used for the colitis brought on systemic lupus erythematosus, a serious immune disorder.

To me this was a case of systematic suppression of symptoms by drugs, without any awareness that things were going from bad to worse. This person had been off work for six months with an ME diagnosis by the time I saw him. One dose of the correct homoeopathic remedy brought instantaneous relief which, when reported to the doctor, was called a coincidence.

Damage by drugs is a serious problem that is not appreciated or understood. If the idea that a person's symptoms are a sign of an underlying problem were accepted, drugs would have no valid use in medical treatment, except in extreme situations – serious, life-threatening, acute illnesses when the pathology has gone too far and death is the most likely consequence.

VACCINE DAMAGE

A child was vaccinated against measles. Within forty-eight hours the child had a fever and a mild convulsion. The mother was concerned and tried to speak about it to the nurse when the child was due for a repeat vaccination. The mother was the quiet, sensitive type, peaceful, caring and loving, but her concerns were dismissed by the nurse as unimportant. The child was revaccinated, had a severe convulsion and is now a permanent epileptic. There was no family history of epilepsy whatsoever.

Doctors are paid extra if they meet their vaccination quotas. This cannot encourage a sensitive, caring environment in which vaccination is evaluated rationally and objectively.

Of course this approach also completely ignores the question of whether vaccination is a good idea anyway. If seems to damage the immune system in many children. It is usually not noticed and may not show up until much later, if at all. The child may prove to be a slow learner or have some behavioural problems but no one ever relates these to vaccination. I believe that vaccination can make recovery from any other illness more difficult throughout adult life. More than 1 per cent of the children I see every year are vaccine damaged.

Vaccinations can create a sort of poisoning and can be 'antidoted' by homoeopathic remedies, sometimes made from the vaccine, provided the damage is not severe.

LIMITS TO RECOVERY – OUR SCATTERED SOCIETY

No trauma would remain if there were enough release processes working to allow it to be resolved. Loving support from relatives and friends is often enough. Many terrible hurts will be resolved with such help whereas a hurt with no support becomes a lifetime trauma.

We have drifted away from supportive styles of living. We used to live in extended families, surrounded by endless uncles and aunts, cousins and second cousins, grandparents and vast arrays of friends in relatively stable communities with a lot of caring and others ready to take over if one particular carer died.

Nowadays parents may change country, location or position in society and the children, as well as the adults, may lose all their friendships. If this occurs frequently, as it often does in military families, it can result in rootless, disconnected children.

We used to live in villages or tribes or other closeknit groups. I hear stories, often from my Indian patients, where the loss of a mother was no more than a passing crisis, as the aunt stepped in and adopted the whole family of children, aided by numerous relatives. It might even have been a turn for the better.

I remember the slums in London where I studied as a student, where whole communities were shifted from tenement houses to vertical concrete blocks. I can only imagine the social devastation that caused. I have treated a great many dysfunctional, deprived families living in high-rise blocks.

By comparison, in Nepal, a country overrun by aid agencies, one project struck me as remarkable. A slum in Kathmandu was rebuilt by taking each house apart and replacing on its original site, but with improvements, which to me seems infinitely preferable – modernization with a heart. The community lived on more healthily because of clean water, drains, toilets, waterproof roofs, electricity, etc., but with the social fabric built up over thousands of years still intact.

It is our small two-parent, two-children families living hours away from other family members, perhaps devoid of any deep friendships through having moved too often during childhood that lay the foundations for lack of care, support and love. There is no grandmother to help with the kids when the mother is sick, no uncle to act as another father figure if necessary, not enough of anything deep, real, solid and reliable. Once this social fabric has gone, it will take generations to repair. This is the situation in the west, one that supports and encourages trauma.

CHAPTER FOUR

Philosophical and psychological aspects

THE NATURE OF BEING HUMAN

What is the difference, I ask my doctor students, between a corpse and a human being? There is a difference, but what is in one and not the other?

I argue that if you do not know the difference, then how can you know whether your treatment is making the person more corpselike or more human? This is the dilemma of the average doctor. Attacking symptoms usually makes us more corpselike, more deeply sick, and speeds our death and dying. That is the problem of not knowing what you are doing.

I find, too, that the difference between a corpse and a human being is not something that has ever occurred to them, nor is it on the teaching agenda at medical school – a surprising omission, one might think!

Homoeopathy teaches that we are a soul energy in a physical energy body: soul and matter. This is a fairly common, if not universal, perception outside the rampant materialism of western society. The soul has various levels and it radiates energy throughout the body, operating upon us through our minds and our feelings.

Mind is will, intention, determination, thoughts; and feelings are zest, love of life, fear, anger, sadness. There is no feeling without thought and vice versa however and no feeling–thought process is without a physical effect. Everything is always *psyche* (in the mind) and *soma* (in the body) or *psychosomatic*, to use that much-abused word.

71

Put simply, our spirit animates our body and brings it to life through the intermediaries of thought and feeling and thus creates action. In a normal, untraumatized state we are vastly intelligent, have a natural zestfulness and thrive on natural challenges. We can create a precisely appropriate spontaneous response to every event. We also enjoy being affectionate, giving and receiving, communicating with one another and co-operating with others. This is the nature of being human.

However it is not the common state of humanity, and this is because something has gone wrong, something that stops us from expressing these innate qualities. It can be seen in repetitive mistakes, failing to respond appropriately to situations, feeling responses that do not match the situation but which constrict us instead, poor communication and non-co-operation. The reason for this is that we have been hurt and are still hurting from a trauma that occurred a long time ago or may be still happening.

What seems to happen is that *when we are feeling hurt our flexible human intelligence stops processing and responding appropriately*. This is a very important point to appreciate as it underpins human malfunction. It is the basis of disease. It is the foundation from which good parenting is possible. It is the basis for understanding the whole human dilemma. These ideas were developed by Harvey Jackins and are graphically explained in *The Human Side of Human Beings*.

Many perceptive authorities now understand disease in terms of a core 'stuckness' or suffering that has to be dissolved, undammed, to create health. Once we are 'stuck', then every time we meet a similar situation, instead of responding appropriately we seem to go into the old malfunction pattern, become distressed again and reinforce the 'stuckness'. This 'stuckness' has thinking, feeling and physical components acting together synchronously and this perpetual reinforcement is what keeps the pattern alive. It becomes part of our posture, our cellular chemistry, our attitudes, our responses, our jobs, our failures, our whole way of being in the world.

J. Konrad Stettbecher, a Swiss psychotherapist, in his brilliant book *Making Sense of Suffering*, confirms much of what I have witnessed myself. He writes:

> An overloading trauma results in damage to the child's primal self congruence and its ability to order experience [to make sense of what happens to it in normal life after that]. The injury is caused by fear and pain eliciting stimuli [e.g. punishment, withholding] to which the child can only react incompletely, if at all, and which he/she cannot adequately integrate into her/his system. Far reaching injuries originate in deformations of personal and historic truths or in the distortion of reality . . . and result in profound insecurities . . . Many real experiences that should have served to develop consciousness must be banished to the unconscious because they cannot be made to correspond with the received, unreal versions of reality.
>
> Difficult birth processes, misguided child-rearing practices and other early traumas are some of the events that have long lasting, devastating consequences in our lives – from fears, anxieties, and continual feelings of unhappiness to rage, violence, and inability to love, obsessive behaviour, and numerous physical symptoms.

If we consider a person as being like a river we can understand this idea more easily. The source is the soul, which exudes vitality in the form of an everflowing spring. This flows through the body and out through our actions, through the pores of the skin and creates our living, the stream of our life.

Somewhere downstream is a dam, created by wrongly processed and stored feelings, so that the flow is dammed up and overflowing the banks. Excess vitality is accumulating and leaking away above the dam and there is only a trickle below. For example, the congestion may be in the heart, causing leaking of pus through acne or an abscess and coldness of hands and feet through poor circulation. Removing the dam will restore the correct flow and harmony.

The nervous system could be likened to groups of people living around the dam. Those above it are sending out flood messages, reporting flotsam, congestion and high water. Those at the dam are saying there is a blockage caused by silting. Those below it are saying there is not enough water to drink or irrigate the fields and the plants are withering away.

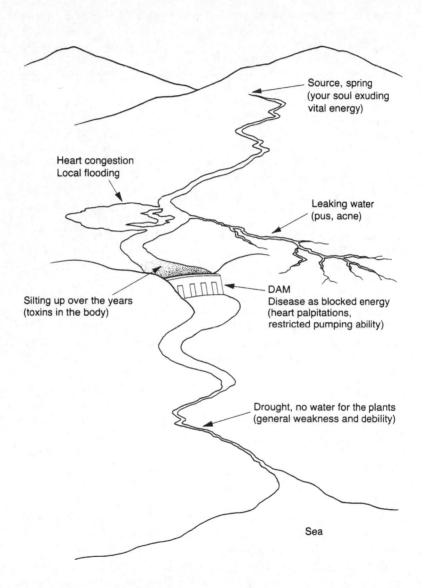

Source, spring
(your soul exuding
vital energy)

Heart congestion
Local flooding

Leaking water
(pus, acne)

Silting up over the years
(toxins in the body)

DAM
Disease as blocked energy
(heart palpitations,
restricted pumping ability)

Drought, no water for the plants
(general weakness and debility)

Sea

Fig. 3 River of life

Taking only one of these messages (as a doctor may do) is clearly wrong. Taking them all as unrelated, as the different consultants in hospitals frequently do (as evidenced by the hospital signposts to separate departments), is clearly nonsense too. The message from upriver of the dam would lead you to think about building higher banks. The downstream message of lack of water might lead you to think the spring had dried up, but the message from the dam itself gives you the vital clue. Taking all the information together allows you to perceive the whole story and even if those at the dam are not sending messages, you can by simple logic deduce that there is a dam.

MAPS OF HUMAN MALFUNCTION

Fortunately homoeopathic remedies are like maps of all known human malfunctions, so one can be found to release the dam, the constriction, and it will be washed away. Initially there will be an increased flow, carrying along with it a lot of debris from the dam and what was accumulated behind it. This is the toxic elimination process which commonly occurs after taking a homoeopathic remedy. Then equilibrium will be restored, all the people living alongside the river will calm down and a sense of peace and harmony will return.

MAINTAINING CAUSES

We have in homoeopathy a concept called a maintaining cause or trauma which perpetuates the problem. A typical example is smoking. If a person has a disease of the nerves like multiple sclerosis, a progressive and slowly developing paralysis, then it is silly for them to smoke and expect to get well. The smoking may be the cause if they developed the disease after starting smoking or it may be a major aggravating factor. So prescribing homoeopathic remedies becomes a waste of time, a collusion between the patient, who maintains the delusion that it is all right to smoke, and the homoeopath who maintains that they are 'doing their best'.

Another maintaining cause is marriages that do not work – and in England that is most of them according to Relate, who are in the best position to know. This means that over half our children are growing up with severely dysfunctional parents who are their role models and yet also the major stresses in their lives.

It seems to me very clear that children need four loving grandparents and two parents who love and respect each other and love and enjoy their children. This is basic common sense. Anything else can fail to provide a proper nourishing environment. If that makes you feel like a less than perfect parent, welcome to the club! As parents, we are all in it together.

Problem solving involves both identifying the problem and doing something about it. Identifying the problem is normally the bit we prefer to skip, hence the problems in western health services. Unawareness of the real cause of our problems – trauma – precludes effective solutions.

EVERYTHING IS REAL

Many problems seem impossible to explain and a variety of reasons is given for their existence; for example, it is God's will, karma, our past lives, bad luck, a genetic mistake. Doctors have likewise invented diagnostic names, abstractions mostly disconnected from reality, which try to explain a complaint when in reality it will have some core trauma behind it.

Doctors are trained primarily to observe, to ignore the patient's peculiarities, to concentrate only on common diagnostic signs which depersonalize, mystify and disempower. My experience is that everything about patients is to be believed on some level, not necessarily at face value but in some way integrated into the picture of who they are. Schizophrenics, for example, hear voices that they cannot block out. In my experience, this is likely to stem from repressed memories of child abuse manifesting as voices in the subconscious. So schizophrenia could usefully be called 'blanked out past thoughts' and this would be helpful in understanding this condition.

These medical names are usually very uninformative to the uninitiated and thus frequently disempowering, leaving the sufferer feeling helpless.

If a person has a problem it is based on real events. Something actually happened to cause it. Perhaps there was trauma in the womb; perhaps the parent wanted desperately to abort the child but changed their mind. What I have seen time and time again is that many severe as well as ordinary behaviour patterns can be explained by something that really did happen, and that if I listen with this in mind, it is frequently revealed to me. I am convinced that underneath all human behaviour are real traumatic events which happened in this life.

When people say their problems stem from past lives I say that may be true but the problem is always reactivated because of traumas re-experienced in this life, even if the initial event occurred in a previous life. With that knowledge you can deal with the problem now rather than letting the suffering continue.

THE ROLE OF THOUGHTS IN TRAUMA

In this book I concentrate on emotional traumas as these are commonly the core of most problems. However, the framework in which we all live includes thoughts, feelings and physical realities, all of which powerfully affect us. And wrong thoughts are often the seed of suffering.

We used to think of illnesses as being caused by germs that attack us, but now holistic medicine understands that blockages and energy depletions encourage toxicity to occur – rather like the muck behind the dam – and germs are just attracted by the mess.

On a larger scale, in my lifetime we have seen the destruction of many thought systems. The Chinese destroyed much of their old cultural heritage, which will have the effect of letting go of old ideas.

Russian communism educated the people and then self-destructed. It was a great thought system but the way it was implemented contained the seeds of its own destruction. By educating everyone from the lowliest peasant it gave people the opportunity to think for themselves and because communist ideas, although good in principle, were implemented in such a crude, ineffective way, it was bound to crumble as the people saw its stupidities.

Historically, people lived in tribes, villages and local areas, fighting over territory, and then graduated to living in nation states governed by kings, but still fighting over territory. We have now had a century or so of fantastic technological advance and aeroplanes, computers, international communications and global organizations are bringing nations closer. Television across borders is now very common and news by satellite is a normal feature of international life. British and American music and American movies with subtitles are teaching whole nations English without effort.

The point I am making is that the pace of change is amazingly fast. The human race is advancing whether it likes it or not, by a process it appears not to comprehend, and old thought patterns have to change more quickly than their adherents might like. Thought systems are being replaced or updated at speed. We seem to have no choice in this. We can only choose whether to become conscious or stay unconscious and although the latter is the more painful path in the long term, most of us take it.

The medical profession in western countries is in this predicament. The basic current medical model is the assumption that disease just happens and must be got rid of, and that it is not caused by the way the person lives. Medicine as widely practised in the west is thus an unconscious thought-based process which makes people sicker, helping to turn their personal crisis into a personal catastrophe and leading to speedier and often more painful deaths.

What we are witnessing in homoeopathic medicine is basically a quantum leap ahead of the current medical consciousness. Homoeopathy is poised to move rapidly to the forefront of medicine, along with a large range of other healing systems, to create a pluralistic comprehensive health care system encompassing the best of the old and the new, where the current monopolistic conventional medicine will be relegated to the roles it performs best – surgery, life saving and physical diagnosis.

In our own lives we also have to develop our thinking.

Frequently when a person takes a homoeopathic remedy it frees them from emotional traumas and fears and by becoming more open, they are able to take in new thoughts. The relative 'stupidity' of previous living becomes apparent and changes take place. We see life more clearly.

Most thoughts are not thoughts at all but feelings dressed up or expressed through the medium of thoughts. They may be powerful feeling–thoughts like the urge to do good, idealism, or negative ones like feelings of inadequacy. Either way, they can arise from deep inner processes based on aspirations and idealism or negative internal feelings. If you examine thoughts closely you will observe that many are basically feelings.

VULNERABILITY AND CAUSATION

Homoeopathy incorporates the idea of vulnerability, which explains why one person is easily affected by an event when others similarly exposed are not. This vulnerability is often rooted in the family life history of the person, and in their parental conditioning, and this often explains the process. Beyond this, it is difficult to appreciate fully but I will attempt to explain.

I would speculate that diseases like tuberculosis were generated from the accumulated debris of repeated 'action replay' traumatization of the entire human race. In simple terms, we made ourselves vulnerable to perfectly normal natural organisms by our crazy behaviour and then called the results diseases. This process took place over long periods of time, as these trauma processes were consolidated and confirmed. Like AIDS, they were a sudden event after a long preparation. Once in existence they can be measured and detected and have the power to reinfect any person vulnerable to them and make them even more vulnerable again.

I am therefore suggesting that all diseases may be the result of human trauma patterns that we made ourselves vulnerable to on a mass level. They should be considered as the final results of our global trauma process and named after them. So tuberculosis could be renamed 'fear in kidneys incarcerating anger of the lungs' and arthritis 'anger stored in joints', which would be much more useful, informative and empowering.

Vulnerability and causation are like the chicken and the egg. There is no first causation or vulnerability, they just are, and each needs the other to exist. They are the tools of the irritation and pain that create crisis and the possibility of consciousness-raising, apparently the main purpose of life.

A NEW LANGUAGE FOR SYMPTOMS

Part of the problem of understanding health and disease is in the words that are used. The more technical they are, the more removed they are from the problem. Frequently medical terms are just synonyms. You go in to see the doctor with earache and come out with otitis media. However, both of these terms bear little relationship to the cause, naming only the effect. Medical names are very disempowering, they make you feel less able to cope with the illness. Nor do they help you cure yourself or prevent it happening again.

To make the underlying process more obvious I think it would be helpful if we gave meaningful names to symptoms so here are some examples.

Eczema   Anger coming out through the skin
Itching   Irritation coming out through the skin
Headaches   Anger exploding in the brain as pain
Vertigo   Being pulled in two directions causing physical imbalance
Inflammations   Local anger toxins incarcerated by fear of being angry
Joint problems   Tension in muscles from anger stored in them, causing tightness and strain on joints leading to excess pressure, inflammation and distortion
Acne   Poisonous resentments showing on the face
Cancer (non-smoking)   Long-held resentments focused into one area
Depression   Unexpressed anger incarcerated by fear, based on known or unknown (pre two years old) causes
Asthma   Anger incarcerated in the lungs by fear held in the kidneys
Eye problems   Inability to see what is in front of you
Ear problems   Cannot or will not hear

Deafness Will not hear, switched off
Stiffness Overcontrol and rigidity on all levels
Sinusitis, hayfever, sneezing attacks, allergic nasal complaints
Unexpressed tears

Even these are only a halfway house and it is much better to define them in a personal way. Once you get the idea I am sure you can invent sensible names for many common problems in your family and friends, which will differ for each individual and not relate particularly to the disease process. 'Mum gave up on Dad years ago and now she is suffering the consequences of suppressing her anger with her bad joints' might be a good example.

INFLAMMATION AND VIRUSES

Flies clear away rotting food. That is their job. Rotting food attracts flies; flies do not attract rotting food. You could, however, be forgiven for being confused if you always saw rotting food and flies together. In medicine this confusion still occurs. Toxicity – local accumulation of poisons – is cleared by germs. It is not the germs that cause the inflammation; they act as dustmen, like the flies, clearing up the mess. Toxicity attracts germs, germs do not attract toxins, and inflammation is a cleansing and healthy process.

MODERN PSYCHOLOGY

From modern depth psychology and homoeopathy has come a simple yet penetrating understanding of trauma and disease. When overwhelming trauma happens we are frozen, wholly or partially, at the age at which it occurs. We act as if we have not developed beyond the stage at which we were traumatized at. Granted we still grow physically but even the height to which we grow can be related to our traumas. Sometimes trauma is so strong and genetics so weak that even our growth is stunted and we do not develop ovaries or testicles fully.

Normally what happens is a partial freezing of our development. Some people pass from childhood to old age without ever becoming adult. In essence they act as children all their lives. They are frozen children in one major or minor aspect of their character.

When we address the trauma with a homoeopathic remedy we bring it to the surface for a subconscious or semiconscious rerun. It becomes an 'action replay' of the old situation with a difference – as if the fears and feelings of the trauma are re-experienced, without the traumatic events. Before you start worrying about what you might go through, however, remember that this is mostly done in our dreams and is rarely noticed on a conscious level.

By bringing the trauma to the surface of our subconscious and rerunning it at a time when we can deal with it, we resolve it and unfreeze the person. They can grow up naturally for the first time or grow back to their old self if that was dented. Frequently after homoeopathic treatment, people report that they feel 'like their old self again'.

If the person was frozen in infancy or earlier, this late growing up will naturally take time; not as long as the actual time lost but usually months and often years. I have seen adult men in their thirties grow up from naively adoring women in an infantile way to a more mature realization of every woman's imperfections and their own and the importance of developing friendships with women.

MORE ABOUT CONSCIOUSNESS

Perhaps the first step towards a deeper understanding of life is the awareness that there are great secrets to life. Not knowing that they exist is a problem, because if you do not know they exist you are hardly likely to go looking for them.

These secrets are hidden where you would least expect to find them and where the common run of logic and reductionist thinking cannot find them. They are 'stored' in the great simplicities, the things that are so obvious we take them for granted. The secrets are too obvious, therefore we do not see them.

Even if you are told them, you cannot hear them if you are not really open, so they do not penetrate. What you hear depends then on your openness, at a deep level. As you grow older you can *choose* to ignore many things as it can be important to focus on a limited field but to be *unable* to hear is a different level of problem; it is due to unconsciousness.

Another great secret of life is that it is a journey from unconsciousness to consciousness on many levels, personal and planetary, with unconsciousness leading to and creating disease and consciousness creating health. We say in homoeopathy that it is the illness or the disease which creates the crisis where consciousness can arise. If the disease is suppressed or removed then the opportunity is lost. If a correct homoeopathic remedy is administered or an appropriate interaction takes place, then consciousness can result. If during the curative process the signs of cure are suppressed then it is likely that the rising of consciousness will be suppressed and later the cure will fail.

This process is well illustrated by Nat mur. You could consider the typical Nat mur person as a teenager who is unable to relate, very vulnerable internally, who suffers disappointment badly as their tears are blocked. They are thus a crisis waiting to happen. Each relationship is doomed to failure as their instinct is to keep secrets. This builds up inner resentments, creates withdrawal and causes the relationship to end, which they cannot cope with. If someone listens to them and they cry, then they can recover, but only to go off and repeat the process. However if Nat mur is given then they will discover spontaneously, by observation or another experience, that sharing secrets helps build closeness, a basic fact of relationships. The Nat mur then brings about a new level of consciousness, about relating in this case, and heals the grief and the pattern of creating grief. This illustrates the idea of healing creating consciousness.

CONCLUSION

This summer I have been moving from country to country conducting homoeopathic seminars as I write this book. A colleague and I have just delivered a dawn-to-dusk seminar over eight days, with patients coming from a wide area. We have heard about unbelievable suffering: systematic beatings and torture, war, severe shock, orphans who had no one caring for them for the whole of their first year, violent and abusive parenting. Some have resulted in serious terminal pathologies, tumours, serious mental states of disassociation. Virtually the whole gamut of human suffering was expressed in the people who gathered in one small isolated village, tucked away on a dry plain, at an unadvertised, supposedly quiet gathering of homoeopaths in training.

Resurrection, passing through the eye of the needle, the developing of consciousness, is to go through these traumas, using our inner awareness. By going through the suffering we transform it into a new level of consciousness to rise again; to become free of pain and of suffering, to release ourselves from the bondage, from the cross of crucifixion in matter, this earthly life experience, to become conscious in the moment.

So I interpret Christ's message as the process of recovering from trauma, from suffering, which is what this book is all about.

PART 2

Homoeopathy for healing

CHAPTER FIVE

Basics of Homoeopathy

This is the briefest of introductions for beginners. More information can be found in the many books on homoeopathy that exist, some of which are listed in the references.

THE INVENTION OF HOMOEOPATHIC MEDICINE

Homoeopathic medicine has been around for nearly 200 years and has evolved over this time from a series of discoveries and inventions by its founder, Samuel Hahnemann, a German doctor disillusioned with medicine in his day. He discovered or recovered several vitally important principles.

Healing is a rational process

The overriding principle, which he formulated at the end of his discoveries, is that healing is a rational process, that there are principles that are essential to guide practice, and that once these are understood then homoeopathy becomes a rational scientific process. We say it is both an art and a science because case taking requires art and human skills, while the actual healing is scientific.

Like cures like

The second principle of homoeopathy is that if a substance causes particular reactions in a healthy person, it can cure an unhealthy person with similar symptoms. For example, peeling onions causes itching eyes and nasal congestion which mimic some people's experience of hayfever. So onion cures hayfever in people who produce these symptoms.

Potentization

The third principle is how poisonous or harmful substances can be rendered harmless yet preserve their curative properties. This could be done, he discovered, by putting them into liquid form (another invention) and then diluting them and shaking them violently, repeating both dilution and violent shaking many times. He called this potentization.

This produced a medically active substance that acted strongly and curatively according to the second principle, yet was free of side effects and very easily made. Nothing like it had been known before. It proved to be alchemy in action, transmuted energy.

The single remedy

Homoeopathy perceives that there is one soul in one body and from this it naturally follows that there is only one core problem at any one time and therefore only one healing intervention, one remedy, is needed to create a curative action. Once this has been done, it is necessary to wait and see what happens before deciding what to do next (although in an acute case this wait might only be a few minutes and one dose might be a frequent repetition over a short period of time).

The whole picture

The single remedy is selected to cover the whole picture of the person since it is the whole person who is sick, not just one part. This principle states that we must consider every aspect of their personal situation, from the widest possible aspects and issues to the smallest and oddest details to get a complete picture.

Hierarchy of symptoms

The principle here is that 'mind' symptoms representing the will, the intentions and the feelings, expressed on many different levels, are usually more important than the physical symptoms. The symptoms can be arranged in a hierarchy, usually of mind over matter, and a remedy is chosen from this perspective, not by looking at the pathology first. (When the major problem is very deeply pathological the mind symptoms may have less significance; for example, in critical heart failure, a heart-focused remedy might be needed, but it would still be based on whole mind–body symptoms.)

Dynamic vitality

This principle says that we are a soul energy vibrating in an energy pattern we call our physical body which is really a vibrational body of energy, vitality, with patterns that keep it flowing in the way we see and experience it. Our soul sends out messages to our mind and these activate energetic feelings and actions of speech, movement, etc.

Disease occurs when there is a conflict between desired action and actual effect owing to dynamic energy blockages. Blockages are maintained by energetic thought, feeling and physical processes and must therefore be cured by energetic processes, here called homoeopathic remedies. There is a vitality attached to every pattern of blockage that must be matched by the remedy vitality to overcome it.

Direction of cure

Details of cures are given in the prescribing section, so here it is sufficient just to state the basic principle.

Cure is a dynamic process with certain well-defined characteristics. Fundamentally, it takes place between the soul and the thought/feeling and physical processes so the direction of cure relates to this. There will be a thought, a feeling and a physical response to cure, and all are important. Theoretically the thought and feeling responses come first so usually we find that inner peace is the first reaction, better energy second and physical curative action last. In reality however, only some aspects will be noticed in any given case.

Physical curative signs generally also flow from the deeper levels, the more recent pathologies, into lesser and older pathologies in a continuum of cure in an order determined by the patient history. Often cure flows from the inside out and from higher up the body to lower down, so from the heart to the joints, from the trunk to the feet, and in respiratory complaints, from the lungs to the nose (up but out) in the reverse order of the progress of the patient's sickness.

Not infrequently the patient relives in a mild form all their previous illness history. For example, one person may relive a few seconds of everything they have ever suffered, spaced a few hours apart; others may have somewhat longer replays of old illnesses.

HOMOEOPATHIC REMEDY SOURCES

Each homoeopathic medicine, or remedy as many homoeopaths prefer to call them, is a very dilute but potentized substance drawn from nature – minerals, metals, plants, and animal and human disease products being common sources. Some are inert in their natural state. Many, such as snake venom, are poisons. They also include toxic metals like mercury and lead, and disease products like gonorrhoea. I say this to remove any misconceptions that homoeopathic remedies are 'gentle, friendly herbs'. They are not. They are powerful, effective healing energies often derived from serious natural poisons, but not given in a poisonous dose.

EVOLUTION OF HOMOEOPATHY

Symptom dictionaries

Further progress has been made in systematizing homoeopathy by categorizing, listing and collating clinical experience. Repertories (symptom dictionaries) which list emotional and physical symptoms have been developed, refined and computerized to great effect (the computerized listings now have over 133,000 headings and subheadings).

Trauma pictures

Gradually it became clear that particular remedies suited certain definable psychological types and specific traumas, which homoeopaths call by various names – remedy essence, materia medica or trauma pictures. Experience has gradually proved that a person fitting an essence or trauma picture and given the appropriate remedy will get better irrespective of what is wrong physically, although in reality mind and body symptoms go together in the patterns described. In other words, all physical symptoms mirror the mind state and vice versa. When accurately perceived, mind states, thoughts and feelings reflect the deepest current trauma or inner state that it is necessary to treat. The inner intelligence of our immune system always presents what is wrong at the forefront of our being, so as to 'request' curative help. Frequently the presentation is based on very early experiences.

Beyond this, homoeopathy has integrated much from the field of modern psychology, both humanistic and traditional, and the importance of conception, birth and early childhood experiences is now recognized by some homoeopaths.

Bringing homoeopathy up to date

It is natural that anything that has existed for a long time becomes out of date, at least in its interpretation, while the basics remain true. This has happened to homoeopathy. Most homoeopathic literature is over a hundred years old and although some of it is still sound, much is a repetition of past dogmas relating to nineteenth-century ways of thinking. Most importantly homoeopathy developed before depth psychology and was thus naive in many respects because of its lack of psychotherapeutic understanding. The cross-fertilization of the two disciplines is now taking place, and this book is I hope, a small step in the process.

TRAUMA PATTERNS

Each homoeopathic remedy has its own distinct picture of what it can cure. Generally speaking, this is in terms of the emotional state of the patient and the unique signs and symptoms of diseases. As an example, the homoeopathic remedy Ignatia (derived from St Ignatia's bean) is suitable for a person who is idealistic, romantic and suffers from grief, losses and disappointments. Ignatia people tend to sigh a lot. This is their 'calling sign', often reflecting tension in the diaphragm (situated below the lungs) which is to do with cutting off feeling from below it. Ignatias tend not to cry easily, and to do so reluctantly and in private. They do not eat fruit and are often scared of feathered and flying things.

All these peculiarities are detailed in the trauma patterns, a mental/emotional/physical susceptibility in a particular direction, the substantial list of peculiarities and mundane facts associated with each remedy. These 'facts' are in reality a deep reflection of the person's inner intelligence, materializing in breathing patterns, in patterns of food likes and dislikes, in patterns of sweating and dryness, in postural and sleeping patterns, in patterns of vocabularies and the specific words and sayings we choose to use, in attitudes, in our jobs and careers and the many other things that discriminate one individual from another.

Many of these patterns are deeply symbolic; for example, Nat mur hates to talk about his or her upsets and has dry lips and dry eyes, i.e. does not express his or her emotions. Likewise the words people use and the clothes they wear are indicative of their trauma. Nat murs use the word 'hate' a lot, while Cannabis types use 'beautiful'; Apis, made from bee sting, may wear black and yellow, even striped, clothes.

TAKING THE MEDICINE

Taking a homoeopathic medicine is easy. They are put into the mouth and absorbed directly through the taste and smell senses into the nervous system.

Remedies are found in tablet form in healthfood shops worldwide, but these reflect a simplified approach, aimed at self-help. Of course, this is better than nothing but the safest and, I believe, the most effective way to take a homoeopathic remedy is by the liquid dose called LM1. This is diluted 50,000 to 1 after initial preparation into solution. You can buy these from specialist homoeopathic chemists. Addresses and phone numbers are given in the Appendix and remedies can usually be sent by post at little cost.

Dosage instructions are given on pages 225–8.

CHAPTER SIX

Homoeopathy for sceptics

In this chapter I address those who remain sceptical about homoeopathy and provide information and ideas that might help them to cross the threshold from disbelief to appreciation. This is not so much a set of well-ordered arguments as a discussion of the most common objections and some of the thoughts and processes which may erroneously sustain disbelief.

A TRANSFORMING EXPERIENCE

My interest in homoeopathy was stimulated by the following experience. Over a ten-year period, my father suffered from gangrene moving slowly up his legs. This necessitated having his legs amputated bit by bit until he died. He had the best medical treatment available, we thought.

My mother remarried and later my stepfather developed a gangrenous ulcer on his leg that needed a district nurse to attend to it three times a week, for years. My first ever prescription, Secale 6x, one pill a day for ten days, cured it completely and for ever. You can imagine the impression that made on me and its symbolism.

THE PLACEBO EFFECT

Many people, especially doctors, knowing that there are virtually no detectable active ingredients in homoeopathic pills, maintain that the results obtained from them must be due to a placebo effect. However, homoeopaths know that this is not true because they commonly give wrong prescriptions (probably every working day, if they are honest). Both the homoeopath and the patient think that they will work, but if they are wrong they do not. In fact we have a saying in homoeopathy that 'the wrong remedy does not work even with the best homoeopath'.

In fact we are highly critical when it comes to validating our prescriptions. We have quite clear criteria for cure (listed in Chapter 10) which spell out what we expect. We often do not obtain the required result, even though the patient may indicate some improvement. Deciding whether the patient is cured or not is a most important aspect of our process, since if we deceived ourselves the whole thing would become farcical. Being critically honest and correct about the effect of a remedy is the key to deciding what to do next.

A BBC film showed a herd of cows which responded to homoeopathic remedies in convincing ways; it is hard to believe that this was due to a placebo effect. In a trial, the incidence of mastitis in half the herd was cut by 95 per cent by using homoeopathic remedies compared to the other half. Babies also respond very well. And rigorous, faultlessly conducted, scientifically controlled, double blind trials show that homoeopathy works well, much better than placebo (Taylor and Reilly; see reference section).

THE INTERVIEW EFFECT

The other common view of homoeopathy is of the interview effect; that it is a long caring interview which makes people better, since it may be the first time the person has ever been listened to. But if it were true that people could be cured just by listening to them, much of what we call medicine would cease to exist. The fact is that even an excellent interview with incredibly sensitive listening and highly skilled interventions will not cure much; otherwise psychotherapists would be miracle workers. However, psychotherapists notice that their clients who visit homoeopaths get through their life dramas much more quickly than clients who do not.

BELIEF MAKES IT WORK

A very common misconception is that you have to believe in homoeopathy for it to work. That is wrong. If you take the correct remedy when it is needed, it will work in spite of you; homoeopathic remedies are stronger than your inhibitions, suspicions and scepticism. As a extremely sceptical ME sufferer said one month after his first prescription, 'If feeling well again and having energy to spare is how you judge success, then I am better, and I have to admit that it occurred within three days of starting your remedy, so the coincidence is hard to ignore.'

SUCCESSFUL PRACTICE

The fact that I have earned my living from practising homoe-opathy for over eighteen years without advertising, just personal referral, is in itself an indication that the system works. People only refer when they find that something works and they do not return when it does not, especially when it costs them good money and the alternative is free.

DOCTORS AS PATIENTS

Nowadays most of my patients are doctors themselves, bringinf me the full gamut of human ailments, and they get better in spite of their occasional scepticism. As one doctor with ME said, 'I was sure your analysis of me and the prescription was wrong and I was still sure it was wrong after a month, but now that I can concentrate my mind again and think more clearly and my energy is returning, I begin to believe it.'

Many of these doctors have complaints of twenty years' standing and they have tried every form of conventional approach to no avail.

PILLS FOR TRAUMA?

Because this book is about using homoeopathy for curing emotional traumas I want to address another common response to homoeopathy: 'How can pills or remedies do anything about emotions?', In other words the concept that you can treat emotional traumas with pills in a holistic and psychotherapeutic way is strange and unbelievable. At best, you might think it is like Valium, hiding the trauma rather than dealing with it.

So what does the homoeopathic remedy do to cure all these long-drawn-out patterns and release all the stuck energy? How can a medicine affect your psychology and mend a trauma from conception or birth or from upbringing? How can a remedy cure lack of loving support?

There is no way I can prove to you that emotional trauma creates physical disease although you might, on reflection, know it to be true from your own experience.

The remedy is based on a substance that has the qualities, found by the principle of provings mentioned before, that resonate with the inner mind-body disease process. It reminds the mind of what is wrong. This is necessary because it has been stuck in this disease pattern for so long it acts as if its normal and the original healing stimulus appears to have almost been forgotten. When a sick person takes a remedy in potentized form it magnifies the symptoms of the disease. This artificially induced reminder automatically creates a new healing stimulus to replace or reinforce the original almost forgotten one. The healing stimulus then mobilizes the normal inner healing process, as if the problem had only just occurred.

WHY IS HOMOEOPATHY STILL NOT BELIEVED?

The question of how homoeopathy works has exercised the minds of scientists for many years but eminent brains, when faced with convincing, scientifically conducted experiments by leading medical researchers reported in leading medical journals such as *The Lancet* and *Nature*, say flatly, 'It can't be true.'

To be realistic, most doctors are too committed to their current belief systems, practices and ways of working to do any more than take a passing interest. In surveys most doctors now say they think homoeopathy is valid, paying lip service to the idea, but few go further than that, although more advanced practices are now offering homoeopathy and other alternatives.

Scientists in general, it seems, are still intolerant of anything that requires them to look beyond accepted safe 'facts'. When I asked a leading scientist to put his mind to this problem, he answered typically, 'It can't be true because you dilute remedies beyond Avogadro's number, but my wife uses them for our children and they seem to work.' In fact the remedies recommended in this book do contain physical quantities of the original substance and so that objection is invalid here.

The now famous scientific experiment devised by Benveniste, a reputable French scientist, and repeated by others over a three-year period on several continents was reported in 1988 in the premier scientific journal *Nature*. It showed that homoeopathic remedies with 'nothing' in them had definite detectable effects. It was immediately derided and scorned, in the *Nature* editorial, in the press and on TV, by an organized 'quack-busting' forum because it confounded established beliefs. I learned from this that people with fixed ideas are not interested in facts and truth, and this includes many scientists.

So ignorance, 'head in the sand' attitudes and a refusal to see are significant reasons why alternative methods of healing are still being sidelined. But science now validates homoeopathic medicines and will surely do so more and more as the trials continue – as indeed is rapidly happening with all forms of alternative healing. Trial after successful trial are showing that energy medicine works and works well. Scientists and mystics are converging and it is now only a matter of time before disbelief dissolves in the face of new knowledge and new facts.

HOMOEOPATHY VERSUS MODERN MEDICINE

Homoeopathy developed initially by experiment, by systematically poisoning teams of healthy people with small doses of the remedies and from here by observations put together slowly and systematically by very able people over a century or two. The facts have converged with time; they have not changed in substance from the beginning.

It is interesting to contrast the longevity and unchanging principles and practices of homoeopathy with scientific medical treatments, where most drugs have a fifteen to twenty year life cycle: five as wonder drugs, five to ten involving increasing side effects, and five being withdrawn or awaiting a replacement; or even worse, remaining in widespread use because the withdrawal effects are too difficult to cope with, as is the case with Valium.

WHAT THEN ARE THESE REMEDIES?

Homoeopathic remedies are not medicines, nor do most of them contain anything significant; yet the action of the remedies can be detected by scientific apparatus. If there is nothing measurable in these homoeopathic remedies (actually all the prescriptions recommended in this book do contain measurable quantities, around 1 in 10,000,000,000,000) and yet they have an effect, what are they?

Let us digress a bit. We all know when we are feeling well or sick or full of energy or low in energy. We can then detect our own energy/vitality level in ourselves yet there is no measurement you can make to show this. There is no meter you can attach to the body to show the energy level. If you go to your doctor feeling weak does he measure you to prove it? Of course not. In fact, you may remember that the great weakness disease now called various names like ME or postviral syndrome was originally called malingerer's disease, as most doctors saw it that way, because they could not measure tiredness and because they were trained not to believe what their patients told them.

Energy

Everything is energy. We ourselves are nothing but energy in patterns of association. Many ancient therapies work with this energy, calling it various names such as *prana* in yoga and *chi* or *qi* in acupuncture. All healing that is holistic works with our own vitality.

Homoeopathic remedies are also patterns of energy and the making of homoeopathic remedies is a way of getting this energy pattern out of physical matter and into a transferable and storable form – something totally remarkable and wonderful in its own right. Each remedy is a specific energy pattern made from an originally physical substance and each one is named after the substance it was derived from. However, after a long process of two hundred years of experiment and developing understanding, they could now justifiably be named after the traumas they address and cure. Since traumas are archetypal human distress patterns which must be as old as humans themselves, these trauma remedies are then the archetypal remedies that address the same patterns of trauma as all other energy therapies. The archetypes appear in the Greek myths, in Shakespeare's plays and in modern psychology. Therapies such as acupuncture, psychotherapy and many eastern-based systems all address these archetypal forces.

So with homoeopathy we are using energies attuned to complex psychological and physical trauma patterns to stimulate and resolve these trauma patterns.

CHAPTER SEVEN

Guidelines for treatment

What I have outlined in this book is a simple yet profound way of healing emotional traumas. These ideas can be applied safely if the guidelines in this chapter are followed and provided you work within your own level of confidence and competence.

Below I attempt to define safe areas for self-help. Obviously if you never knew birth traumas existed, you are not going to know what you are doing when you try to resolve them, especially if they happened many years ago. But if you are trying to help a recently born baby the situation may be clearer. Common sense has to be applied to the guidelines.

Jung, that sage of psychotherapy, has a saying which is relevant here to the effect that the healer never comes alone. This implies that some more spiritual or other guidance will take place along with your good intentions and actions.

HELPING YOURSELF

Do not. We say a self-prescriber has a fool for a prescriber and an idiot for a patient. Get someone else to help you unless you are very objective. If you find that several trauma pictures fit you then more external help is needed, a friend perhaps. If only one fits neatly then perhaps you are correct in your prescription but who will support you in the curative process? Find a friend for support − you deserve it.

GENERAL GUIDELINES

1. Only try helping with problems you feel some confidence in dealing with. Start with very easy situations and gain your skills slowly and carefully within your limits.
2. Start with situations where the problem and solution are very clear:

- People with only one problem, e.g. a grief, a stress or a disappointment that can be easily understood;
- Infants and children who are mostly well;
- People without a disease;
- People with disorders that are not serious, like temporary headaches, and where death is not a possibility;
- People who have not led complex and traumatic lives;
- People who have lived satisfactory lives without chronic illness but have run into one overwhelming trauma;
- People who have been to the doctor and found that the tests show nothing really wrong;
- People for whom there is no more than one disease in the history of the family, e.g. tuberculosis in only one grandparent.

3. If the situation is not clear, or you feel uncertain or lacking in confidence, then you should seek professional help. *If for any reason you are not certain and confident as to what to do then you should not proceed.* This would be asking for trouble. If you are cautious and have been successful in previous situations using the remedies as directed then you could try something a bit more difficult.
4. If you are of an impulsive disposition then you should rein yourself in and stop trying. If you reach beyond your capacity you could cause difficulties that you may not be able to resolve.

WHERE PROFESSIONAL HELP IS NEEDED

1. People who are diagnosed as ill, mentally or physically;
2. People on any drugs, whether prescribed or not;
3. People with a compulsion or addiction, such as alcoholics, compulsive gamblers etc. Compulsions are normally the

after-effects of severe traumatization, often as an infant, and are not easy to resolve;

4. People who do not want to be helped, if they are old enough to say so;

5. People with something that has been going on for many years, unless it is superficial;

6. People with symptoms that have been successfully stopped by drugs or creams, e.g. severe rashes that are fully under control;

7. Asthmatics;

8. Old people lacking vitality or wanting to die;

9. Very old people;

10. People with many diseases in their family history. I know that this rules out lots of people but these are more difficult cases and not for beginners.

HELP SHOULD BE REQUESTED

Help should only be given to those people who request it or who are in your care. My experience is that you should never break this rule because unwilling participants who do not positively request help but only try it because you want them to will find ways of sabotaging the help given and will frustrate the process. If you are someone who always wants to help people, this is called being a rescuer. It is an addiction and you should attend to it before helping others as it can mask your judgement. Homoeopathy requires unprejudiced observation, not compulsive helping.

PEOPLE WITH OTHER MEDICAL OR THERAPEUTIC SKILLS

I hesitate to be too restrictive here, as it depends on the situation, and the availability of professional homoeopaths. There is no doubt in my mind that homoeopathy can complement and enhance many other therapeutic intervention processes and make them more effective. But doctors, for example, find it very hard to prescribe so little. They often confuse their homoeopathy by frequent repetition and thereby get it wrong. My experience is that other therapists should stick to the above guidelines until they have *good reliable experience*. Many fail to master homoeopathy simply because they start with the most difficult situations.

TREATING THE TRAUMA OR THE PERSON

Sometimes the trauma seems obvious at first, but may not be so later, and you may be in a quandary. For example, a person may seem like Nux vomica yet be suffering from grief like Ignatia. The answer here is to take what is most clear and obvious in the person. If they are still acting like a Nux vomica in grief then give that. If they are clearly now acting like an Ignatia, give that. When it is difficult to decide, giving the trauma remedy first is a safer option.

TAKING THE CASE

Understanding the patient

'Case' is a word we use to cover understanding and listing everything wrong with a person. Obviously in some cases you will know all the facts but it is still a good idea to write them all down and arrange them in order. Consider the friend or family member to be helped. What do you know for certain about them? Talk to them about their life. Listen between the lines, not to the facts but to how they express them. What are the critical events? How did they respond to these events? Often a spouse, parent or friend can help fill in gaps or even get together as a group to pool ideas.

What are the repeating sagas of their lives? How do they face the world? What were their parents' biggest problems? Have these been handed down? What fears, attitudes and other facts are definite? Why did they choose their particular job and their spouse. Why did they have children?

To understand these things, write down all the facts and then think about them. Sit with them in silence and try to put yourself in the position of the person you are trying to help by feeling what it must have been like. This is a powerful way to appreciate the problem. Do not go just by the facts, as often it is the response to an event that you need to understand, not the event itself. Events only indicate possibilities, not reality.

Keep it all as simple as possible, sticking to the minimum solid reliable facts and your strong gut feelings (unless you are an impulsive person, when your strong gut reactions may say more about you than the other person; this is a very common mistake – you must know yourself!). One or two really strong and certain facts are better than ten disputable ones.

When you are satisfied that you have a good reliable short-list of facts, story lines, etc., go to the indexes. By going through each index, you may spot things that are strongly linked to the friend you are helping. At this point an interactive understanding may take place between the helper and the helped, translating ideas into homoeopathic clues, clarifying an agreed 'right feeling' about the situation, and relating these clues through the indexes to possible trauma pictures.

I find this an important step. When I discuss with a patient how I see their life and one or both of us modify our views, we rapidly converge on the truth and get to the point where we agree. Then I feel sure that we are on the right track.

Having generated a shortlist of possible indexes and, from these, remedies that stand out, check each one and reach a definite conclusion, choosing one remedy.

A word of warning. You can easily read yourself into any number of the indexes and remedies, so remember that the facts should be very strong if you are treating yourself. If you are helping someone else, then it is easier to be objective. The first disease of homoeopaths is to think they are the remedy they have just learned about and to take it.

Analysis in detail

Make a written list of what you know for certain about the person – causation, attitudes, food preferences, fears, etc., as in the indexes.

Then consult the indexes and write down the ones that correspond. In cases where there is no exact correspondence, be careful not to use something that is not true. Consult the person and see if the index seems correct to them; if you cannot find one to correspond, ignore this quality rather than approximate.

Copy out all the indexes that fit the person and the listed remedies onto a piece of paper; about five indexes would be a good maximum.

Now look at the whole list and see if any remedies are represented in all or most of the indexes. Ideally one remedy, or perhaps two or three, should be strongly represented. Be especially guided by the main remedies indicated by the type-face. This process gives you a selection of possible remedies, one of which should suit the person.

Then go to the trauma patterns and see if one fits well. Combinations of remedies are not an option.

If after considerable effort you cannot fix on one remedy there are lots of possible reasons:

1. Only the most common remedies are listed here. It could be another, but this is unlikely.
2. The person you are trying to help may be much more complex than can be understood without professional training.
3. The information in the indexes is restricted to try to keep it manageable and this may have excluded what you need.
4. Some people appear very different externally from what they are inside.
5. Pathological information is very limited here and some people go straight from trauma to pathology without the clues in between.

Example 1

Let us assume that the subject has suffered a broken love affair.

Love, disappointed: AUR, *Bell*, *Caust*, HYOS, *IGN*, Kali c, *Lach*, NAT M, Nux v, PH AC, Phos, Sep, STAPH, Sulph, Tarant.

We also know that their nails are always very short and we can see them biting them, so:

*Biting nails, pulling hair out: ACON, ARS, *Bar c*, Calc, Carc, Caust, *Hyos, Lyc, Med, Nat m*, Nit ac, Phos, Puls, *Sil*, Staph, *Stram, Sulph, Tarant*.

From living with them we know they definitely dislike fatty things:

Dislike fats and rich food: *Ars*, *Bell*, *Calc*, *Carc*, CHINA, Lyc, *Merc*, NAT M, Nit ac, Phos, PULS, *Sep*, *Sulph*, Tarant.

They dislike high places because they make them giddy:

High places, vertigo: ARG N, Aur, CALC, *Nat m*, Phos, Puls, Staph, SULPH.

They often sleep on their front and it is the position they feel most comfortable in:

Sleep on front: Ars, *Bell*, Calc, *Carc*, Caust, *Coloc*, Ign, Lach, *Lyc*, MED, *Nat m*, *Phos*, PULS, *Sep*, *Stram*, *Sulph*, *Tub*.

We see from the above that Nat mur occurs five times out of five, Pulsatilla four times out of five, Sulphur five out of five, etc. If we give a score of 4 for bold italic capitals, 3 for capitals, 2 for bold italic and 1 for plain typeface (see key on p. 111) we can make a simple sum to see which is most strongly indicated, as this method gives a more exact emphasis. Thus we get Nat mur 12, Sulphur 10 and Pulsatilla 9. However, we must also consider the strength of the symptom in the person; for example, if we are absolutely convinced that disappointment is the cause we can rule out Pulsatilla. So numerical sums should not overrule gut reactions as to what is important.

Having derived a shortlist of possibilities, Nat mur, Sulphur and Pulsatilla, we then go to the trauma patterns. We soon discover that Sulphur is itchy, untidy and philosophical, while Pulsatilla is soft, weepy and yielding and Nat mur is close, reserved, dry, sheds few tears and is vulnerable, and we can quickly decide which of these best fits the person in question.

Example 2

Here a woman has been badly upset by her daughter-in-law and is very angry but cannot express it. She feels humiliated and suffers from indignation at the wrong done to her. One other well-known thing about her is that her hair went grey early.

Anger, suppressed: *Aur*, Carc, Cham, *Ign*, LYC, *Nat m*, Sep, *STAPH*.

Humiliation with indignation: *STAPH*.

Hair, goes grey: *Ars*, LYC, *Nat m*, *Ph ac*, *Sil*, *Staph*, *Sulph*, Thuja.

Here the only remedy is Staphisagria. If you read the trauma pattern you can see that these people are subservient, sweet-natured and a victim type which fits very well with what you know.

Example 3

This young teenager has had hayfever ever since a tuberculosis vaccination. The root of her nose is blocked. Everything else is normal. She likes company and does not like being alone. She is thirstless and dislikes heat and crowded rooms, need-ing fresh air. She cannot eat fat of any description – she hates it. She used to have a strong fear of dogs which she has now overcome.

Dislike of fats and rich food: *Ars*, *Bell*, *Calc*, *Carc*, CHINA, Lyc, *Merc*, NAT M, Nit ac, Phos, PULS, *Sep*, *Sulph*, Tarant.

*Company, desire for: ARG N, ARS, *Calc*, HYOS, *Ign*, KALI C, LYC, *Nux v*, *PHOS*, *Puls*, *Sep*, STRAM.

Fear of dogs: *BELL*, *Calc*, Carc, *Caust*, CHINA, *Hyos*, Lach, Merc, Nat m, Plat, *Puls*, Sep, Sil, *Stram*, Sulph, TUB.

A shortlist derived from these shows Calcarea (5), Pulsatilla (7) and Sepia (5) and a check of the trauma patterns for these three shows that she is clearly Pulsatilla.

COMMON QUESTIONS

Here are the answers to some of the most common types of questions I am asked.

1. *If I have a person who has most of the characteristics of one trauma pattern but not the pathology, can it be the remedy?*
Yes, if the pattern fits it can cure any problem.

2. *I know someone whose main keynote is being very talkative. Could they be Lachesis? Nothing else fits – or I do not know about others, so could I try it?*
No. This would be guesswork and very unreliable. There are lots of loquacious remedies.

3. *I have a friend who is part Sepia and part Pulsatilla. Can I try both together or one after another?*
No. The friend can only be one remedy at one time; they are one soul in one body, with one problem requiring one solution. Wait until you have more information. Study both remedies and think up questions which could decide it one way or the other. In this example, information on thirst or the effect of heat or dancing would help.

4. *I have read all the pictures and I found bits of me in several of them. Could I try one and if so, which?*
This is a common problem of homoeopathic students. As I said before, in this situation you have a fool for a prescriber and an idiot for a patient, unless you are very thorough, so it is necessary for you to find someone else to help you.

ONE FINAL AND IMPORTANT SUGGESTION

Prescribe only when you feel certain of the remedy. If you are not sure study longer, collect more information, get one of the books recommended, seek extra help, do anything but prescribe. If you follow this golden rule you will have wonderful results and as your experience grows you will be able to do more. Treat it like driving in a new place. First you use the main roads with large signposts to get around. As you become confident you try the side road and discover more routes as you get your bearings.

So go slowly at first and send people you cannot figure out to someone who can.

CHAPTER EIGHT

Indexes of Remedies

HOW TO USE THE INDEXES

These are to be used as guides to finding the correct homoeopathic remedy for the trauma you are trying to heal. A range of indexes is included to give you various entry routes into the remedy system.

It is important to be flexible: not to miss obvious things like the job a person does, but at the same time to look at the crisis they are now experiencing, as this may reflect everything about the person. Some things will reinforce each other: a mental rigidity, a stiff back and a stiff finger for example all point at the same idea. These things are important.

Different typefaces are used for the remedies to indicate different degrees of importance in relation to a particular sign or symptom. This information is backed up by almost 200 years of clinical experience, so it is reliable.

Ordinary typeface means the remedy is indicated for this sign or symptom.

Bold italic upper and lower case means the remedy is more commonly indicated for this sign or symptom.

CAPITALS means the remedy is a *key* note; commonly used for this sign or symptom.

BOLD CAPITALS IN ITALICS means it is the *top* remedy for this sign or symptom.

So the short form for this is

TOP, KEY *Common*, indicated

Sometimes the indicated remedies are omitted for the sake of

111

simplicity, as may be the common remedies and this is shown by an asterisk * in front of the sign or symptom.

Homoeopaths please note that these listings do not conform exactly to existing homoeopathic literature because some remedies have been deliberately highlighted when they are well known clinically in relation to a symptom, although current literature may not reflect this. The information comes from the Complete Repertory of Roger van Zandvoort, published electronically at present in MacRepertory (see Appendix 1 for details), and I am very grateful to Roger for masterminding this twenty-first century repertory and for permission to use it and extract from it.

LIST OF REMEDIES

Acon	Aconite
Anac	Anacardium
Arg n	Argentum nitrate
Arn	Arnica
Ars	Arsenicum
Aur	Aurum
Bar c	Baryta carbonicum
Bell	Belladonna
Calc	Calcarea carbonicum
Cann i	Cannabis indica
Carc	Carcinosin
Caust	Causticum
Cham	Chamomilla
China	China
Coloc	Colocynthis
Hyos	Hyoscyamus
Ign	Ignatia
Kali c	Kali carbonicum
Lach	Lachesis
Lyc	Lycopodium
Med	Medorrhinum
Merc	Mercury
Nat m	Natrum mur
Nit ac	Nitric acid
Nux v	Nux vomica
Ph ac	Phosphoric acid
Phos	Phosphorus
Plat	Platina
Puls	Pulsatilla
Sep	Sepia
Sil	Silica
Staph	Staphisagria
Stram	Stramonium
Sulph	Sulphur
Tarant	Tarantula hispania
Thuja	Thuja
Tub	Tuberculinum

KEY TO THE INDEXES

TRAUMA CAUSATION INDEX

In using this index, you should look for the main causation – the one that best describes the trauma. You may see other headings that are applicable and these may also help, but you should select only the main one.

Be careful when deciding on the best description; weigh it up thoroughly. Sometimes it is easy – there is only one remedy for ailments from recent disappointment, for example – Ignatia. Betrayal, on the other hand, gives many possibilities.

Sometimes the cause and the attitude may coincide. For example, the cause may be jealousy, and the general attitude may also be jealous. At other times the cause may be jealousy, but the person may not normally be jealous. It may therefore be necessary to differentiate two similar positions, and I have tended to group similar headings together to help with this differentiation.

It is important to remember that this section is all about causation.

TRAUMA CAUSATION INDEX (THE STRESSES)

ANGER CAUSATION

Anger, suppressed: *Aur*, Carc, Cham, *Ign*, LYC, *Nat m*, Sep, *STAPH*.

Anger with indignation: Ars, *Aur*, COLOC, Lyc, Merc, Nat m, *Nux v*, Plat, *STAPH*.

Anger with silent grief: *Acon*, Ars, Aur, Bell, Carc, Cham, *China*, *Coloc*, Hyos, IGN, LYC, *Nat m*, Nux v, *Ph ac*, Plat, Puls, STAPH.

Contradiction, being told off, deeply traumatized by this: Anac, *Aur*, Cham, *Ign*, Med, Sil.

Code: *TOP*, KEY, *Common*, Indicated

Humiliation, shame, being put down forcibly, something that is too hard to bear: *Acon*, Anac, *Arg n*, Ars, *Aur*, Bell, Calc, CHAM, *COLOC*, IGN, Lach, LYC, Merc, NAT M, *Nux v*, PH AC, Plat, *Puls*, *Sep*, *Sil*, *STAPH*, Stram, *Sulph*.

Humiliation with anger: *COLOC*.

Humiliation with indignation: *STAPH*.

*Offence, taking: *Acon*, ARS, *Aur*, Bell, CALC, *CARC*, CAUST, *Coloc*, Lach, LYC, *Med*, *Nat m*, *Nit ac*, NUX V, *Plat*, *Puls*, *Sep*, *Sil*, STAPH, *Sulph*, *Thuja*, TUB.

Offences from the past: Calc, *Cham*, *Ign*, *Staph*.

Punishment; person, typically a child, becomes ill from punishment: *Ign*, Nat m, Tarant.

Reproaches, being censured with severity, severe language (see Humiliation): Bell, Carc, Coloc, *Ign*, Med, *NAT M*, Nux v, Ph ac, Plat, *Staph*, *Stram*, Tarant.

Rudeness of others: Anac, *Calc*, Carc, Med, Nat m, Nux v, Ph ac, STAPH.

Scorn, being scorned, subject to extreme and passionate contempt: Acon, *Aur*, Bell, CHAM, *Coloc*, Hyos, Lyc, *Nat m*, NUX V, *Phos*, *Plat*, Sep, *Staph*, Sulph, Tarant.

Violence: Aur, Sil, STRAM, Tarant.

FEAR CAUSATION

*Anticipation, stress, exam nerves, stage fright, nerves before appointments, etc: *Anac*, ARG N, ARS, *Bar c*, CALC, CARC, *Caust*, China, Hyos, IGN, LYC, MED, Nat m, *Ph ac*, *PHOS*, *PULS*, *SIL*, *Tub*.

Embarrassment: Coloc, *Ign*, Ph ac, Plat, Sep, Staph, SULPH.

Fear: ACON, Arg n, *Bell*, Calc, Carc, *Caust*, *Ign*, Lyc, Phos, Puls, *Sil*.

*Fright: ACON, *Arg n*, *Aur*, *Bell*, *Calc*, CAUST, *Hyos*, IGN, *Lach*, LYC, NAT M, *Nux v*, PH AC, PHOS, *Plat*, PULS, *Sep*, SIL, *Stram*.

Fright from sight of an accident: *ACON*.

Code: *TOP*, KEY, **Common**, Indicated

GRIEF, LOSS, BETRAYAL CAUSATION

Betrayal: AUR, Ign, Lach, LYC, Merc, NAT M, *Nux v*, Ph ac, Puls, Sep.

Betrayal of ambition: Bell, Merc, *Nux v*, Plat, Puls.

Betrayal of friendship: Ign, Nux v, Ph ac, Sil, Sulph.

Death of a child: Calc, CAUST, *IGN*, Lach, Nat m, Nux v, Ph ac, Plat, Staph, Sulph.

Death of parents or friends: Ars, Calc, CAUST, *IGN*, Nit ac, Nux v, Plat, Staph.

Disappointment: Acon, Ars, AUR, CAUST, *Cham*, *Coloc*, Hyos, *IGN*, *Lach*, LYC, *Merc*, NAT M, *Nux v*, PH AC, Plat, PULS, Sep, *STAPH*.

Disappointment, new: *IGN*.

Grief: Anac, *Arn*, AUR, *Bell*, *Calc*, *Carc*, CAUST, *Coloc*, *Hyos*, IGN, LACH, NAT M, *Nux v, PH AC, PHOS, Plat, Puls*, SEP, Sil, STAPH, Tub.

Grief, and cannot cry: Carc, *Ign*, NAT M, Nux v, Puls.

Grief, recent: Ign.

Homesickness: *Ign*, PH AC.

Love, disappointed: AUR, *Bell*, *Caust*, HYOS, *IGN*, Kali c, *Lach*, NAT M, Nux v, PH AC, Phos, Sep, STAPH, Sulph, Tarant.

Love, with silent grief: IGN, NAT M, PH AC, Phos.

MISCELLANEOUS CAUSATIONS

Alcoholism: Ars, Calc, Lach, Nux v, Ph ac, Sulph.

Bad news: *Arn*, CALC, *Cham*, *Coloc*, *Ign*, *Med*, *Merc*, *Nat m*, *Nux v*, *Staph*, *Sulph*.

Business failure: Calc, Coloc, Nat M, Nux v, Ph ac, Puls, Sep, Sulph.

Discords between chief and subordinates: Lach, Merc, Nat m, Nit ac, Nux v, Sulph.

Discords between parents, friends: Ars, Lach, Merc, *Nat m*, Nit ac, Nux v, Sulph.

Domination by others, long history of: Carc, Lyc, Sep.

Code: *TOP*, KEY, *Common*, Indicated

Excitement, emotional: *Acon*, *Arg n*, *Aur*, *Bell*, *Calc*, *Caust*, IGN, *Nat m*, *Nux v*, PH AC *Phos*, PULS, *Sep*, STAPH, *Tarant*, TUB.

Excitement sexual: *Nat m*, *Plat*, Staph.

Horror, sad stories, ghost stories: *Aur*, *CALC*, *Caust*, *Lach*, *Lyc*, *Nit ac*, *Nux v*, PHOS, *Puls*, *Sep*, *Sil*, STAPH, *Sulph*.

Hurry: *Acon*, *Arn*, *Nit ac*, Nux v, *Puls*, Sulph.

Isolation: *Anac*, *Arg n*, Cann i, Plat, Puls, *Stram*.

Jealousy: *Hyos*, *Ign*, *Lach*, NUX V, *Phos*, PULS, Staph.

Joy, excessive: *Acon*, Ars, Aur, Caust, China, Mere, Plat, Caust, *Puls*.

Literary or scientific failure: Calc, Ign, Lyc, Nux v, Puls, Sulph.

Money, loss of: *Arn*, *Ars*, Aur, Calc, *Ign*, Nux v, Puls.

Position, loss of: *Ign*, *Plat*, Staph.

Pride, traumatized self-importance: *Calc*, *Lyc*, Merc, Sil, *Sulph*.

Quarrels: Thuja.

Rage, fury: *Arn*, *Aur*.

Rejection, abandonment, desertion, (compare Isolation): Anac, *Arg n*, AUR, Bar c, Calc, Cann i, Carc, China, Kali c, *Lach*, *Merc*, *Plat*, PULS, Sep, *Stram*.

Reverses of fortune: Lach, Staph.

Sexual abuse: see Chapter 3.

Sexual celibacy, no sexual outlet: Phos.

*Sexual excesses: CALC, CHINA, *Kali c*, LYC, *Merc*, NUX V, PH AC, PHOS, *Puls*, SEP, *Sil*, STAPH.

Shame: see Humiliation, Indignation, Sexual abuse, Offence, Contradiction, Embarrassment.

Shock: see Fright.

Stress: see Anticipation.

Surprises, pleasant: China, Merc.

*Work, mental: *Anac*, *Arg n*, *Kali c*, *Lach*, *NUX V*, *Ph ac*, *Sil*, STAPH, *TUB*.

Code: *TOP*, KEY, *Common*, Indicated

ATTITUDE, BEHAVIOUR AND PERSONALITY INDEX

These are to do with the natural way a person is, things about them that stand out strongly that can be taken as a guide to selecting their homoeopathic remedy. Sometimes headings seem similar, such as Impetuous and Impulsive. Some of the remedies for these will overlap and some will be different. It may be important to consider which is most appropriate.

The most important thing is only to use the person's definite attributes: those that several people would agree on. If someone always gulps down their food and finishes before anyone else, this is definitely hurry in eating.

Sometimes you can assess a person's attitude by the words they use – words such as 'hate', 'resent', 'isolated' or 'rejected'. Or they may speak abruptly, or talk in revolutionary terms. These things should be noted and used where appropriate to decide on their attributes.

ANGER, EXTERNALIZED ONTO OTHERS

Abruptness of manner: *Calc*, Cham, Lyc, Med, Nat m, Nit ac, Nux v, *Plat*, PULS, Sil, Sulph, *Tarant*.

*__Abusive, insulting:__ *Acon*, *Anac*, *Arn*, *Aur*, *Bell*, CHAM, *Hyos*, *Ign*, LYC, *Nux v*, *Sep*, *Stram*, Tarant, Tub.

Abusive, children insulting parents: Hyos, Lach, Lyc, Nat m, PLAT.

Anarchism: Arg n, Caust, Merc.

Anarchism, revolutionary: *Caust*, Kali c, MERC, Sep.

Bitterness, exasperation: Ars, Ign, Nit ac, Puls, Sulph.

Blaming of others: ACON, ARS, Aur, *Calc*, *Carc*, Cham, Caust, CHINA, *Hyos*, Ign, *Lach*, *Lyc*, Med, *Merc*, *Nat m*, *Nux v*, Sep, *Staph*, Sulph.

Break things, desire to: *Bell*, Hyos, *Nux v*, Staph, *Stram*, Sulph, Tarant, *Tub*.

*__Contemptuousness:__ *Arg n*, *Ars*, *China*, *Lyc*, *Nux v*, PLAT.

Code: *TOP*, KEY, *Common*, Indicated

Contradiction, disposition to: ANAC, *Ars*, *Aur*, CAUST, LACH, *Lyc*, *Merc*.

*****Criticalness:** *Arn*, ARS, *Bar c*, *Caust*, *Lach*, *Lyc*, *Nux v*, *Phos*, *Plat*, *Sep*, SULPH.

Cruelty, inhumanity: *ANAC*, *Ars*, Bell, Carc, China, *Hyos*, *Lach*, Med, *Nit ac*, Nux v, *Plat*, Staph, *Stram*, Tarant.

Cruelty, to animals: ARS, Bell, Calc, Med.

Destructiveness: *Bell*, Calc, Carc, *Hyos*, Lach, *Nux v*, Phos, Plat, Staph, *STRAM*, Sulph, *Tarant*, Tub.

Enemy, considering everybody: *Merc*.

Estrangement from family: Anac, Arn, Ars, *Nat m*, *Nit ac*, Nux v, Phos, Plat, *Sep*, Staph.

Hardheartedness, lack of feeling, cold hard look: *ANAC*, Ars, Hyos, *Lach*, Plat, *Sulph*.

*****Hatred:** ANAC, *Aur*, *Calc*, *Cham*, *Lach*, *NAT M*, *Nit ac*, NUX V, *Ph ac*.

Hatred, of men: Bar c, Ign, Lyc, Phos.

Hatred, of women: Puls.

Kill, desire to: Anac, *Ars*, Bell, Calc, China, HYOS, Lach, *Lyc*, *Med*, Merc, *Nux v*, *Phos*, *Plat*, Sil, *Staph*, Stram.

Mocking: Acon, Ars, China, Hyos, Ign, *Lach*, Nux v, Plat, Tarant.

*****Quarrelsomeness:** *Anac*, *Arn*, *Ars*, AUR, *Bell*, *Caust*, *Cham*, *HYOS*, IGN, *Kali c*, *Lach*, *Lyc*, *Merc*, *Nat m*, *Nit ac*, NUX V, *Ph ac*, *Phos*, *Plat*, *Sep*, *Sil*, *Staph*, *Stram*, SULPH, *TARANT*, *Thuja*.

*****Rage, fury:** *Acon*, *Anac*, *Arn*, *Ars*, BELL, HYOS, *Lach*, LYC, *Merc*, *Nat m*, *Nit ac*, *Phos*, *Puls*, STRAM, *Sulph*.

*****Resentment, revengefulness and maliciousness:** *Acon*, *ANAC*, ARS, *Aur*, *Bell*, *Calc*, *Cham*, *Hyos*, *Lach*, *Lyc*, NAT M, *Nit ac*, NUX V, *Ph ac*, *Staph*, STRAM, TUB.

Ridicule, tendency to: Acon, Hyos, Lach, Nux v.

*****Rudeness:** *Anac*, *Cham*, *Chin*, HYOS, LYC, *Nux v*, *Phos*, PLAT, *Stram*.

*****Swearing:** *Ars*, *Bell*, *Hyos*, *Lyc*, *Nat m*, NIT AC, *Nux v*, *Tub*.

Sympathy, lack of: Anac, Ars, Cham, China, Nat m, Nit ac, Plat, Puls, Sep.

Code: *TOP*, KEY, *Common*, Indicated

ANGER INTERNALIZED AS SADNESS, ETC.

Bad luck, feeling of: Carc, *China*, Kali c, *Lyc*, *Sep*, *Staph*, Sulph.

*Biting nails, pulling hair out: ACON, ARS, *Bar c*, Calc, Carc, Caust, *Hyos*, *Lyc*, *Med*, *Nat m*, Nit ac, Phos, Puls, *Sil*, Staph, Stram, *Sulph*, *Tarant*.

Biting objects: BELL, Hyos, Sil, STRAM.

*Depression, despair: *Acon*, *Anac*, *Arg n*, ARS, AUR, CALC, *Cann i*, *Caust*, *China*, IGN, *Lach*, LYC, *Med*, *Merc*, *Nat m*, *Nit ac*, *Nux v*, *Puls*, *Staph*, *Stram*, SULPH.

*Depression, suicidal disposition from: *Anac*, *Ars*, *AUR*, *Bell*, *Calc*, Carc, *China*, *Hyos*, *Ign*, *Lach*, *Med*, *Merc*, *Nat m*, *Nux v*, *Puls*, *Sep*, *Stram*.

Despair, caused by pain: Acon, *Ars*, AUR, Calc, *Cham*, *China*, IGN, Lach, Med, NAT M, Nux v, Stram.

*Despair, of recovering: *Acon*, ARS, CALC, *Ign*, *Med*, MERC, *Nit ac*, *Sep*.

*Despair, religious: *Arg n*, ARS, AUR, *Calc*, LACH, *Lyc*, *Med*, PULS, *Stram*, *Sulph*, *Thuja*.

Disgust, feeling of: *Kali c*, *Merc*, PULS, *Stram*, SULPH.

Doubt: Ars, Aur, Bar c, Chin, *Lach*, Nux v, Sep, Sil, Staph, Thuja.

*Guilt: ARS, *AUR*, *Bell*, *Caust*, *Hyos*, *Ign*, *Lach*, *Med*, *Merc*, *Nat m*, *Nux v*, *Ph ac*, *Puls*, *Sil*, *Stram*, SULPH, Thuja.

Hanging, suicidal disposition: ARS, Aur, *Bell*.

Killed, desire to be: *Ars*, Bell, Stram.

Sadness, suicidal disposition: AUR, Calc, Caust, China, Ign, Med, *Nat m*, Sep, STAPH, Sulph.

Self-blame: *Acon*, Anac, *Ars*, *Aur*, *Hyos*, *Ign*, Lach, Lyc, Med, Merc, *Nat m*, *Puls*, Sil, Stram, Sulph, *Thuja*.

Self-pity: CALC, Nit ac, *Staph*.

Seriousness, earnestness: ARS, *Aur*, *Chin*, *Merc*, *Staph*.

Smiling, never: ARS, AUR.

Throwing oneself from a height, suicidal disposition: Anac, *Arg n*, Ars, AUR, BELL, Hyos, Ign, Lach, *Nux v*, Sil, Staph, Stram, Sulph, Thuja.

*Weariness with life: ARS, AUR, *Bell*, CHINA, *Merc*, NAT M, *Nit ac*, *Nux v*, *Ph ac*, PHOS, *Puls*, *Sil*.

Code: *TOP*, KEY, *Common*, Indicated

CHAOS

*Chaotic, confused behaviour: *Ars*, *Bell*, CHIN, *Merc*, NUX V, *Ph ac*, *Phos*, *Puls*, *Staph*.

Dirtiness, unwashed appearance: Lach, Med, Merc, Nux v, Phos, *Plat*, SEP, Sil, STAPH, *SULPH*.

Untidiness: Carc, Sil, SULPH.

RUSHING

*Hasty speech: *Bell*, HYOS, *Ign*, LACH, *Med*, MERC, *Ph ac*, *Sep*, *Stram*, *Thuja*.

*Hasty, ejaculation: Calc, *Chin*, LYC, *Nat m*, *Ph ac*, *Phos*, *Plat*, *Sep*, *Sulph*.

*Hurry, always in a great hurry: *Arg n*, ARS, *Aur*, *Bar c*, BELL, *Hyos*, IGN, Kali c, *Lach*, MED, MERC, NAT M, NUX V, *Puls*, SIL, *Stram*, SULPH, TARANT, *Thuja*.

*Hurry, while eating: *Bell*, CAUST, *Lach*, *Plat*.

*Hurry, while walking: ARG N, *Sulph*, TARANT, *Thuja*.

*Impatience: CHAM, IGN, Med, NUX V, SEP, SIL, *Sulph*.

*Impetuousness: *Anac*, *Cham*, *Kali c*, *Med*, *Nat m*, NIT AC, NUX V, SEP, *Staph*, *Sulph*.

*Impulsiveness, sudden desire to do something: ARG N, *Ars*, *Aur*, IGN, *Med*, PULS.

*Run, tendency to, rather than walk: *Bell*, *Calc*, *China*, HYOS, STRAM, *Sulph*, *Tarant*.

*Thoughts, rush of: *Ars*, BELL, Calc, Chin, *Ign*, *Kali c*, LACH, *Nux v*, *Ph ac*, PHOS, *Puls*, *Sil*, *Sulph*.

CONTROL

*Carefulness, taking great care with everything: *Ars*, *Aur*, *Bar c*, CHINA, *Ign*, *Lach*, *Lyc*, *Nux v*, *Sep*, STRAM, SULPH.

Cautiousness: Ars, Bar c, Calc, Caust, Hyos, *Ign*, Nux v, *Puls*, Stram.

Exacting, tendency to be too: *Puls*.

Code: *TOP*, KEY, *Common*, Indicated

*Conscientiousness about trifles: **ARS**, **Bar c**, IGN, **Lach**, **Lyc**, **Med**, **Nux v**, SIL, STAPH, **Stram**, **Sulph**, THUJA.

Tidiness: **Anac**, Arg n, **ARS**, Aur, CARC, **Kali c**, Med, **Nat m**, **Nux v**, Phos, Plat, Puls, Sep, Sil, Sulph, Thuja.

POSSESSIONS, MONEY AND TRUST

Bargain, disposition to: **Puls**, **Sil**, Sulph.

Beg, entreat, tendency to: Ars, Aur, Bell, Kali c, Plat, Puls, Stram.

Dishonesty: Ars, **Hyos**, **Lach**, NAT M, **Tarant**.

Greed, for money and possessions: **Ars**, Calc, **China**, **Lyc**, Merc, **Puls**, **Sep**, Staph, Sulph.

Hoarding: **ARS**, **Lyc**, **Med**, **Ph ac**, PULS, **Sep**, SIL, **Sulph**.

Squandering: **Bell**, Calc, Caust, MERC, **Nux v**, Stram, Sulph.

Stealing: BELL, **Nux v**, **Sulph**.

*Trust, lack of, suspicion: ACON, ANAC, **Arn**, ARS, **Aur**, BAR C, **Bell**, CANN I, CAUST, **Hyos**, LACH, **LYC**, **Med**, **Merc**, **Nit ac**, **Nux v**, **Phos**, PULS, **Sep**, **Staph**, STRAM, SULPH.

PSYCHIC SENSITIVITY

Clairvoyance, psychic sensitivity: Acon, Anac, Arn, Calc, **Cann i**, Carc, Hyos, Lach, Med, **Phos**, Sil, Stram, Tarant.

SELF-ESTEEM, LOW

*Childish behaviour: **Arg n**, BAR C, **Ign**, **Ph ac**, **Stram**.

*Confidence, lack of: **ANAC**, Aur, **Bar c**, **China**, **Kali c**, **Lyc**, **Med**, **Nat m**, **Ph ac**, **Puls**, SIL.

*Cowardice: **Acon**, **Arg n**, **Bar c**, **Cham**, **China**, LYC, **Nux v**, **Puls**, **Sil**, STRAM.

Flattery: Arn, LYC, Nux v, Plat, Puls, Sil, Staph.

Helplessness, feeling of: Anac, Arg n, LYC, Phos, Puls, Stram.

*Indecision, great: **Anac**, **Arg n**, **Ars**, BAR C, **Calc**, IGN, LACH, **Lyc**, **Merc**, **Nat m**, **Nux v**, **Phos**, PULS, **Sep**, **Sil**, **Sulph**.

Code: **TOP**, KEY, **Common**, Indicated

Isolation, feeling of: *Anac, Arg n, Cann i, Plat, Puls,* STRAM.

*Mildness, meekness: *Acon,* ARN, ARS, *Calc,* CARC, *Ign, Lyc,* NAT M, *Nit ac, Nux v, Phos,* PULS, *Sep,* SIL, *Stram, Sulph, Thuja.*

Rejection, abandonment, desertion, feeling of: Anac, *Arg n,* AUR, Bar c, Calc, Cann i, Carc, China, Kali c, *Lach, Merc, Plat,* PULS, Sep, STRAM.

Reverence for others: Hyos, Nat m, Nux v, Plat, Puls, Sil, Sulph.

Servility, obsequiousness, submissiveness: Anac, Lyc, PULS, Sil, Sulph.

*Shyness: *Acon, Ars, Aur,* BAR C, CALC, *Caust, China, Ign,* KALI C, LYC, *Merc, Nat m, Nit ac, Nux v,* PHOS, *PULS,* SEP, *SIL, Staph, Stram,* SULPH, *Tub.*

*Shyness, with poor eye contact: *Bar c, Calc, China, Ign, Merc,* PULS, *Staph, Stram, Sulph.*

Spinelessness: Bar c, *Calc, Sil.*

Success, lack of, expectation of failure: *Arg n,* Aur, Merc, Nux v, Sil.

Yielding disposition: *Ars, Ign, Lyc, Nux v,* PULS, *Sil,* Staph, Sulph.

SELF-ESTEEM, INFLATED

Boasting, bragging: Arn, Ars, Bell, Lach, Merc, Nat m, Nux v, Plat, Stram, Sulph.

Hypocrisy: Bar c, Caust, Lyc, Merc, Nux v, Phos, Puls, Sep, *Sil, Sulph.*

Bossiness: ARS, *Lyc.*

Eccentricity: *Bell, Cann i,* LACH, *Tarant.*

Exaltation of politics: Bell, *Caust,* Lach, Nux v.

Egotism: Anac, Arn, Aur, *Calc, Lach, Lyc,* Med, Merc, Nux v, Phos, PLAT, *Sil,* Staph, Stram, *Sulph.*

Haughtiness: *Caust, Hyos, Lach,* LYC, PLAT, *Puls, Sil, Staph, Stram,* SULPH.

Power, love of: Ars, Lach, *Lyc,* Nux v, Sulph.

Pride: Arn, Ars, Caust, Chin, Hyos, LACH, Lyc, Nux v, PLAT, Staph, Stram, Sulph.

Code: *TOP,* KEY, *Common,* Indicated

Presumptuousness: Arn, Calc, *Lyc*, Plat, Staph.

Selfishness: Ars, Bell, *Calc*, China, Ign, Lach, Lyc, Med, Merc, Nat m, Nux v, Phos, Plat, *Puls*, Sep, Sil, *Sulph*, Tarant, *Tub*.

HAPPINESS, SUPERFICIAL

*Cheerfulness, happiness, not related to actual events: CANN I, HYOS, LACH.

Idealism: *Caust*, *Ign*, *Lyc*, *Plat*, Tub.

Jokiness: *Ars*, *Cann i*, *Hyos*, *IGN*, *Lach*, *Stram*, *Tarant*.

Laughter, immoderate: Anac, Bar c, Bell, CANN I, *Hyos*, Ign, *Nat m*, Nux v, *Plat*, Stram, Tarant.

Laughter, involuntary: Aur, Bell, CANN I, Hyos, IGN, Lyc, *Nat m*, *Nit ac*, Phos, Puls, Sep, *Tarant*.

Laughter, over serious matters: *Anac*, Arg n, Cann i, Ign, Lyc, *Nat m*, Phos, *Plat*, Sulph.

Laughter, during sleep: Bell, Caust, *Hyos*, LYC, Ph ac, Sep, *Sil*, *Stram*, SULPH.

Singing: Bell, *Hyos*, *Lach*, *Plat*, *Stram*.

Singing, loud: *Hyos*, *Stam*.

Smiling: Ars, *Bell*, HYOS, Nux v.

Verses, rhymes and songs, writing or speaking in: *Cann i*, China, Lach, Lyc, Nat m, Staph, *Stram*.

ACTIVITIES, BETTER FROM

Dancing: Carc, Caust, *Ign*, *Nat m*, SEP, Sil.

Music: AUR (classical), Carc, Merc, Nat m, *TARANT* (fast, break dancing, pop), Thuja (church), Tub.

Music, to relieve restlessness of extremities: TARANT.

*Occupation, diversion, inability to watch TV without other activity: Ars, Aur, Calc, Carc, Chin, *Ign*, Lach, Lyc, *Nux v*, Puls, SEP, Sil, Stram.

*Company, desire for: ARG N, ARS, *Calc*, HYOS, *Ign*, KALI C, LYC, *Nux v*, *PHOS*, *Puls*, *Sep*, STRAM.

Code: *TOP*, KEY, *Common*, Indicated

RELIGION

*Doubt of soul's welfare: ARS, AUR, LACH, PULS, *Sulph*.
Fanaticism: Caust, Med, Puls, Sulph, *Thuja*.
Mania: *Lach*, *Plat*, *Puls*, *Stram*, Sulph.
*Religious nature: *Arg n*, *Ars*, *Aur*, *Bell*, *Calc*, *Cham*, HYOS, Ign,
   LACH, Lyc, *Med*, *Plat*, *Puls*, SEP, *STRAM*, SULPH.

JEALOUSY

Envy, desire for what others have (not the same as jealousy): ARS,
   Calc, *Lach*, Lyc, Nux, v, *Plat*, *Puls*, Sep, *Staph*, Sulph.
Jealousy: Anac, Ars, Calc, Coloc, *HYOS*, Ign, Kali c, *LACH*, *Lyc*,
   Med, Nat m, NUX V, Ph ac, *Plat*, *Puls*, Sep, *Staph*, *Stram*, Thuja.

SEXUALITY

Indecent dressing, stripping, streaking, nudism: Bell, *HYOS*, Merc,
   Phos, *Stram*, Tarant.
*Lust: *Acon*, *Calc*, *Cann i*, *Caust*, *China*, HYOS, LACH, PHOS,
   PLAT, *Puls*, *Sep*, *Sil*, STAPH, *Stram*, *Tarant*, *Tub*.
*Sexually amorous disposition: *Bell*, *CALC*, CAUST, CHINA,
   Colc, *Hyos*, IGN, *Lach*, LYC, *Merc*, *MED*, *Merc*, NAT M, NUX V,
   PHOS, PLAT, PULS, *Sep*, SIL, *Staph*, STRAM.
*Sexually lecherous disposition, leering: *Calc*, *China*, *Hyos*, *Lach*,
   Lyc, Med, *Nat m*, Plat, *Sil*.

THOUGHTS

Absorbed in thought: *Arn*, *Nat m*, *Nux v*, *Puls*, SULPH.
*Brooding, dwelling on past disagreeable events, holding grudges:
   Cham, *China*, *Lyc*, *NAT M*, *Plat*, *Sep*, *Sulph*.
*Introspection, meditativeness: ACON, *Aur*, *China*, IGN, *PULS*,
   Sep, SULPH.
Narrow-mindedness: Bar c, Puls.

Code: *TOP*, KEY, *Common*, Indicated

One-track mind: *Ign*, *Sil*.

Philosophy, ability for and tendency to: Anac, Lach, Nit ac, Sulph.

Plans, making many: Anac, Arg n, CHINA, Nux v, Sep, *Sulph*.

Repetitive thoughts: STRAM.

*Theorizing: *Aur*, CANN I, *China*, *Lach*, *Sep*, SULPH.

*Tormenting thoughts: *Ars*, *Caust*, *Lach*, *Lyc*, NAT M, *Nit ac*, *Sulph*.

CONCERN

Injustice, cannot support: Calc, CAUST, Ign, Med, Merc, Nat m, Nux v, Phos, STAPH, Sulph.

Inquisitiveness: Aur, Hyos, Lach, Puls, Sep, *Sulph*.

*Kindness, sympathy: Carc, *Caust*, *Ign*, *Med*, *Nat m*, *Nit ac*, *Nux v*, PHOS.

*Sentimentality: IGN, *Nat m*, NUX V, *Phos*, *Puls*, *Sulph*, *Tub*.

*Worry, anxiety about friends at home: *Phos*, *Sulph*.

*Worry, anxiety about others: *Arg n*, *Ars*, *Carc*, CAUST, *Nux v*, *Phos*, *Staph*, *Sulph*.

INDIFFERENCE

In company, in society: ARG N, Kali c, Lyc, Nat m, *Plat*.

*To business: *Arg n*, *Arn*, *Ph ac*, *Puls*, *Sep*, *Stram*, *Sulph*.

To loved ones, relatives: *Acon*, Ars, Bell, Carc, Merc, *PHOS*, *Plat*, *SEP*.

To opposite sex: *Puls*, SEP, Thuja.

To personal appearance: SULPH.

To welfare of others: Ars, Caust, Lach, Nat m, *Nux v*, Plat, SULPH.

GUARDEDNESS

*Reserve: *Calc*, *Hyos*, *Ign*, *NAT M*, PHOS, *Plat*, *Puls*, *Staph*.

Code: *TOP*, KEY, *Common*, Indicated

Secretiveness: Aur, *Bar c*, Caust, *Ign*, Lyc, *Nat m*, Nit ac, Phos, *Sep*, *Thuja*.

OPENNESS

Extroversion: Acon, Arg n, Bar c, Carc, *Lach*, Lyc, Med, Nux v, *Phos*, Sulph, Tarant.

Naivety: *Bell*, Stram.

Naivety with great intelligence: *China*, Hyos, *Stram*, *Sulph*.

SPEECH

Gossip: Ars, Calc, Caust, Hyos, Lach, Stram.

*Sighing: *Aur*, *Cham*, *IGN*, *Nux v*, *Ph ac*, *Puls*, *Sep*, *Stram*.

*Talkativeness, or tendency to voluminous letters: *Aur*, *Bell*, *Cann i*, HYOS, *LACH*, *Phos*, STRAM.

WILFULNESS

*Courage: *Ign*, *Puls*, *Tub*.

Optimism: *Calc*, Lyc, Nux v, Puls, Sil, *Sulph*, Tub.

*Stubbornness, obstinacy: ANAC, *ARG N*, BAR C, BELL, CALC, CHAM, NUX V, TARANT, TUB.

*Stubbornness, obstinacy in children: CALC, *Carc*, *Cham*, *China*, TUB.

*Work, compulsion to: AUR, *Bar c*, *Carc*, Hyos, *Ign*, *Lach*, *Lyc*, NUX V, *Sep*, TARANT, TUB.

LACK OF WILL

Ambition, loss of: Arg n, Ars, Caust, *Sep*.

*Laziness, especially about work: CHINA, LACH, NAT M, *NIT AC*, NUX V, PHOS, PULS, SEP, *SULPH*, TUB.

Will, divided: ANAC, *Lach*.

Code: *TOP*, KEY, *Common*, Indicated

Will, loss of, lack of drive: Bar c, *Calc*, Lyc, *Merc*, *Nat m*, Phos, *Sil*, Sulph.

Will, weakness of: *Anac*, Ars, *Bar c*, CALC, Caust, China, Ign, Kali c, *Lach*, *Lyc*, Merc, Nat m, Nux v, Puls, Sil, Staph, Sulph, *Tarant*.

FEARS AND PHOBIAS INDEX

Fears are usually ordinary things that a person may be particularly afraid of. As homoeopathic clues they should be strong and definite.

Accident, to a friend: Ars, Caust.

Aeroplanes: *Acon*, Arg n, Ars, CALC, Nat m.

*Alone, being: ARG N, ARS, HYOS, KALI C, LYC, PHOS, *Puls*, *Sep*, *Stram*.

Alone, being, at night: Arg n, *Caust*, *Med*, STRAM.

Alone, being, lest he die: *Arg n*, ARS, *Kali c*, *Phos*.

Alone, being, and deliberately injuring himself: Ars, Merc, Sulph.

Animals: BELL, Calc, Carc, Caust, CHINA, Hyos, Lyc, Med, Nat m, *Stram*, TUB.

Animals, imaginary: *BELL*.

Birds: Ign, NAT M.

Black: Ars, STRAM, Tarant.

Blind, becoming: *Nux v*, *Sulph*.

Brilliant objects, mirrors, etc: Cann i, Lach, Stram.

Burglars (looks under the bed for them): Anac, *Arg n*, ARS, Aur, Bell, *Ign*, *Lach*, Lyc, *Merc*, NAT M, *Phos*, Sil, Sulph.

Busy streets: *Acon*, Bar c, Carc, Caust.

Cancer: ARS, Bar c, CALC, *Carc*, Ign, Med, Nat m, *Nit ac*, Phos, PLAT, Sep.

Cars, travelling in: Acon, Arg n, *Aur*, *Lach*, *Sep*.

Cats: Calc, China, Med, *Tub*.

Cemeteries: Stram.

Church or theatre, when ready to go: ARG N.

*Claustrophobia: *Acon*, *Arg n*, *Calc*, *Ign*, LYC, Med, PULS, STRAM.

Code: *TOP*, KEY, *Common*, Indicated

Contagion: Bar c, CALC, *Lach*, Sil, SULPH.

Corners, walking past certain: *Arg n.*

Creeping, something creeping out of every corner: Med, *Phos.*

Crossing a bridge: Arg n, Bar c, Puls.

Crowds, public places, agoraphobia: Acon, *Arg n*, *Arn*, Bar c, Nux v, Puls.

Cruelties, excited by report of: Calc.

Dark: *Acon*, Arg n, Ars, Bell, *Calc*, CANN I, Carc, Caust, China, Hyos, *Lyc*, *Med*, Nat m, *Phos*, *Puls*, Sil, *STRAM*, Sulph, Tub.

*Death: *ACON*, *Arg n*, *Arn*, *ARS*, *Bell*, CALC, *Cann i*, *Caust*, *Kali c*, *Lach*, *Lyc*, Med, *Merc*, *Nat m*, NIT AC, *Nux v*, *Ph ac*, PHOS, PLAT, *Puls.*

*Death, when alone: *Arg n*, *Arn*, ARS, *Kali c*, Med, *Phos.*

Dentist: Calc, Puls, Tub.

Disabled, becoming: ARS.

Disasters: *Puls*, *Tub.*

Doctor: Arg n, Arn, Ign, Nat m, *Nux v*, *Phos*, *Sep*, *Stram*, *Thuja*, *Tub.*

Dogs: *BELL*, Calc, Carc, *Caust*, CHINA, *Hyos*, Lach, Med, Merc, Nat m, Plat, *Puls*, Sep, Sil, *Stram*, Sulph, TUB.

Enemies: Anac, Hyos.

Evil: *Arg n*, *Ars*, CALC, *Caust*, *China*, *Lach*, *Nat m*, *Phos*, *Sep*, *Staph*, *Stram.*

Failure: Arg n, Arn, Carc, Lyc, Nat m, Phos, Sil, Sulph.

Fainting: *Acon*, *Arg n*, *Plat.*

Falling: Acon, Arg n, Ars, Calc, Caust, China, Kali c, Med, Nux v, Phos, Sil, *Stram*, Tub.

Ghosts: *Acon*, *Ars*, Bell, Calc, Cann i, Carc, *Caust*, China, *Hyos*, Kali c, *Lyc*, Med, *Phos*, *Plat*, *Puls*, Sep, *Stram*, *Sulph.*

*Happening, fear that something will happen: Ars, *Calc*, CAUST, *Coloc*, *Nat m*, NUX V, *Ph ac*, PHOS, *PLAT*, TUB.

Happening, something terrible: *Ign*, *Sep.*

Heart disease: Acon, Arg n, *Arn*, *Aur*, *Calc*, *Caust*, Lach, *Med*, Nat m, *Phos*, Tarant.

High places, vertigo: *Arg n*, *Aur*, Calc, Carc, Nat m, Phos, Puls, Staph, Stram, *Sulph.*

Code: *TOP*, KEY, *Common*, Indicated

Humiliation: Puls, *Sep*.

Imaginary things: *Acon*, Ars, BELL, Lyc, Merc, *Phos*, Sep, STRAM.

Injury: Arn, Ars, Aur, Cann i, China, Hyos, Kali c, STRAM.

*Insanity: ANAC, *CALC*, CANN I, *Med*, *Merc*, *Nat m*, *Nux v*, *Phos*, PULS, *Sep*, *Staph*, *Stram*.

Insects: CALC, Lyc, Nat m, Phos, Puls, Sulph.

Job, losing: Calc, Ign, Puls, Sep, Staph, Sulph.

Knives, (keep them out of sight): Ars, China, Hyos, Merc, Nux v.

Late, being: *Arg n*, Med.

Lightning: Bell, Lach, Phos, Sil.

Looked at, being: ARS, Bar c, Calc, *Cham*, *China*, Merc, *Nat m*, Nux v, Sil, Stram, Sulph, Tarant, Thuja, *Tub*.

Men: Acon, Anac, *Aur*, *Bar c*, Bell, Ign, Lach, *Lyc*, Merc, *Nat m*, Phos, *Plat*, *Puls*, Sep, Sulph.

Music: *Acon*, Bar c, Nit ac, Nux v, Phos, Sulph, Tarant, Thuja.

*Noise, general: *Aur*, *Bell*, *Caust*, *Cham*, *Lyc*, *Med*, *Phos*, *Sil*.

Noise, from rushing water: Hyos, STRAM, Sulph.

Noise, at night: Bar c, *Caust*.

Noise, at door: *Aur*, *Lyc*.

Noise, from street: Bar c, *Caust*.

Observed, one's condition being: CALC.

Ordeals: *Arg n*, Arn, Ars, Thuja.

*People: *Acon*, *Anac*, *Aur*, *Bar c*, *Caust*, HYOS, *Kali c*, LYC, *Nat m*, *Plat*, *Puls*.

People, in children: BAR C, *Lyc*.

Periods, during: Acon, *Bell*, IGN, *Lach*, *nat m*, Nux v, *Ph ac*, Phos, Plat, Staph, Sulph.

Pins, sharp things: Ars, Merc, Nat m, Plat, SIL.

Poisoned, being (a specific form of suspicion): Anac, *Ars*, *Bell*, *Hyos*, Ign, *Lach*, Nat m, Ph ac, Phos.

Poverty, worry over money: ARS, *Calc*, Kali c, Nux v, Puls, *Sep*, Staph, Sulph.

Public, appearing in: Anac, Arg n, *Lyc*, SIL.

Self-control, losing: *Arg n*, Cann i, *Merc*, Nux v, *Staph*, Sulph, Thuja.

Code: *TOP*, KEY, *Common*, Indicated

Shadows: *Calc*, Phos, Staph.

Sleep, going to: Calc, *Lach*, Merc, Nat m, Nux v.

Snakes: Arg n, *Bell*, *Carc*, *LACH*, Nat m, Puls, Tub.

Someone behind them: Anac, Lach, *MED*, Merc, Staph.

Spiders: Calc, Carc, Nat m, Stram, Tarant.

*****Stomach, 'butterflies' in:** ARS, *Aur*, *Bar c*, *China*, *Kali c*, *Sulph*, *Tarant*.

Strangers: *Bar c*, Carc, Caust, Lach, Lyc, Puls, Sil, Stram, *Thuja*, Tub.

Streets, busy: *Acon*, Carc, Caust.

Strangled, being: PLAT.

Struck, being, by people coming towards them: ARN, Bell, Ign, Kali c, Lach, Stram, Thuja.

Subways, underground: ACON, STRAM.

Suffocation: ACON, *Ars*, Lach, Merc, Nux v, *Phos*, *Staph*, *Stram*, *Sulph*.

Suffocation, at night: Arn, Ars, *China*, *Lyc*, Med, *Puls*, Sil, *Suph*.

Suicide: Arg n, *Ars*, Lach, Med, *Merc*, *Nux v*, Plat, Sep, Tub.

Thunderstorms: Bell, *Calc*, Carc, Caust, *Coloc*, Lach, Lyc, *Merc*, *Nat m*, *Nit ac PHOS*, *Sep*, Sil, STAPH, Stram, Sulph, Tub.

*****Touch:** *Acon*, *Arn*, *Bell*, *Cham*, *China*, *Kali c*, *Nux v*, *Tarant*.

Tunnels: *Ãcon*, Arg n, Bell, Nat m, *STRAM*.

Undertaking anything: *Arg n*, *Ars*, *Llyc*, Nux v, Sil.

Violence: see Injury, Struck, Burglars.

Water: *Bell*, Cann i, Carc, HYOS, *Lach*, Med, Merc, Nux v, *Phos*, STRAM, Sulph, Tarant.

Wind: *Cham*, Thuja.

Women: Puls, Sep, Staph.

Work: *Arg n*, Calc, Cham, China, Coloc, Hyos, *Kali c*, Lyc, Nat m, *Nux v*, Phos, *Puls*, *Sil*, *Sulph*.

FOOD LIKES AND DESIRES INDEX

Food likes and dislikes reflect three things: the person's natural inner intelligence, searching out what's best for the bodily needs

Code: *TOP*, KEY, *Common*, Indicated

and nutrition; food fads ingrained through outside influences; the person's social conscience, for example being vegetarian because you dislike the way animals are kept.

The preferences given below are the *natural preferences*, not those resulting from fads or social influence. So if you usually eat what you believe is good for you, try to forget this here and choose only those things that strongly reflect what you would really like, irrespective of its origins or whether it is good for you or not. If you love meat or ice cream or fat but do not eat them, they are still valid.

Only choose something if it is strong and certain.

*Alcoholic drinks: *Arn*, *ARS*, *Aur*, *Calc*, *China*, LACH, *Lyc*, *Med*, NUX V, *Phos*, *Puls*, *Sep*, *Staph*, SULPH, *Tub*.

Bananas: Thuja, Tub.

Bitter drinks: NAT M, Sep.

Bitter food: *Nat m*, Nux v, Sep.

Bread: *Ars*, *Aur*, *Bell*, Cann i, *Cham*, *Coloc*, Ign, Lyc, Merc, *Nat m*, *Puls*, Sil, Staph.

Bread, and butter: Bell, Ign, MERC, Puls.

Bread, rye: *Ars*, *Ign*.

Butter: Carc, Ign, Merc, Nit ac, Puls, Sulph, Tub.

Cheese: *Arg n*, Calc, Carc, Caust, Ign, *Nit ac*, *Phos*, Puls, Sep, Tub.

Chicken: *Phos*.

Chocolate: Arg n, *Calc*, *Carc*, China, Lyc, Nat m, *PHOS*, Puls, *Sep*, Sulph, Tarant.

Coffee: Arg n, *Ars*, *Aur*, Bell, Calc, Cham, *China*, Lach, NUX V, Puls, Sulph.

*Cold food: *Ars*, *Cham*, *Ign*, *Lyc*, *Merc*, *Nux v*, PHOS, PULS, *Sil*, *Thuja*.

Cucumbers: *Phos*, *Sulph*.

*Delicacies, sweet and spicy titbits: *Aur*, CHINA, TUB.

Eels: *Med*.

Eggs: *Calc*, *Carc*, Caust, *Puls*, Sil, Tub.

Eggs, hard boiled: CALC.

Eggs, soft boiled: *Calc*, *Puls*.

Farinaceous food, pasta etc: *Calc*, *Carc*, Lach, *Nat m*, *Sulph*.

Code: *TOP*, KEY, *Common*, Indicated

Fat: Arg n, Ars, Calc, *Carc*, *Med*, Nat m, NIT AC, *Nux v*, Phos, Sil, *Sulph*, *Tub*.

Fat ham: *Carc*, *Tub*.

Fish: Caust, *Med*, *Nat m*, *Nit ac*, Phos.

Fish, salty: *Nat m*.

Fish, herring: NIT AC, *Puls*.

Fruit: Ars, *Carc*, *China*, *Ign*, Lach, Med, Nat m, PH AC, Phos, Puls.

Fruit, acid: *Ars*, Calc, China, Ign, Lach, Thuja.

Fruit, Green: Calc, *Med*.

Hot food: Ars, *LYC*, *Ph ac*.

Ice : Arg n, *Ars*, *Calc*, *Med*, Phos, Sil.

Ice cream: Arg n, *Calc*, Carc, *Med*, *Nat m*, PHOS, *Sil*, Sulph, Tub.

Indigestible things: *Aur*, Bell, *Calc*, Ign, LACH, Nat m, NIT AC, SIL, Sulph, *Tarant*.

Juicy things: *Ars*, China, Med, Nux v, PH AC, Phos, Puls, Staph.

Lemonade: BELL, Calc, Lach, *Nit ac*, Puls.

Lemons: Ars, BELL, *Merc*, Nat m, Puls, *Tarant*.

Lime: *Calc*, Hyos, Ign, Nat m, NIT AC, *Nux v*, Sil, Sulph, *Tarant*, Tub.

*Meat: *Calc*, *Nux v*, *Staph*, *Sulph*.

Meat, pork: Nit ac, Nux v, *Tub*.

Meat, raw: *Phos*.

Meat, smoked: *Carc* CAUST, TUB.

Milk: Anac, *Ars*, *Aur*, *Calc*, *Carc*, *Lach*, *Merc*, *Nat m*, *Nux v*, *Ph ac*, *Phos*, *Sil*, *Staph*, *Sulph*, Tub.

Milk, cold: Carc, *Ph ac*, *Phos*, Staph, *Tub*.

Olives: Calc, LYC, Sulph.

Onions, raw: Carc, Med, Staph, *Thuja*.

Oranges and orange juice: MED.

Oysters: *Calc*, LACH, *Lyc*, *Nat m*, Phos, *Sulph*.

Pepper: Carc, *Nat m*, Nux v.

Pickles: Ars, Ign, *Lach*, *Sep*, Staph, *Sulph*.

Potatoes: Calc, Med, Tub.

Raw food: Calc, Ign, Med, SIL, SULPH, Tarant.

Code: *TOP*, KEY, *Common*, Indicated

Refreshing things: *Ars*, *Calc*, *Caust*, *China*, *Med*, *PH AC*, *Phos*, *Puls*, Thuja, *Tub*.

Rice: Phos, *Staph*.

Salty things: ARG N, *Calc*, *Carc*, *Caust*, *China*, *Med*, *NAT M*, NIT AC, *Ph ac*, PHOS, Sil, Staph, Sulph, *Tarant*, *Thuja*, *Tub*.

Sauces: Arg n, *Nux v*.

Seasoned food, highly: Acon, Arg n, *Ars*, Aur, Carc, Caust, CHINA, Nat m, Nit ac, *Nux v*, *PHOS*, Puls, Sep, Staph, SULPH, *Tarant*, Tub.

Soup: Carc, Merc, Nat m, *Staph*, Sulph.

*Sour foods, acids: ACON, ARN, *Ars*, *Calc*, *Cham*, *China*, *Ign*, *Kali c*, *Lach*, *Med*, *Nat m*, Ph ac, *Phos*, *Puls*, Sep, *Stram*, SULPH.

Strange things during pregnancy: Calc, *Sep*.

Sugar: ARG N, *Calc*, Carc, Kali c, *Lyc*, *Phos*.

*Sweet things in general (not the same as chocolate): ARG N, ARS, *Calc*, CANN I, *Carc*, CHINA, *Kali c*, *LYC*, *Med*, *Merc*, *Nit ac*, *Phos*, *Puls*, *Sep*, STAPH, SULPH, *Tub*.

Tea: Thuja.

Tomatoes: Ign.

Vegetables: Ars, Cham, *Sulph*.

Vinegar: Arn, Ars, Carc, *Nat m*, Puls, *Sep*, Sulph.

Wants something but does not know what: Cham, *China*, IGN, *Lach*, PULS, Sil.

Warm drinks: ARS, Bell, Carc, Kali c, *Lyc*, *Sulph*.

Warm food: ARS, *Lyc*, Med, *Ph ac*, Sil.

FOOD DISLIKES AND AVERSIONS INDEX

These are things you really do not like, *not* what you do not eat because it is bad for you or it is cruel, nor because the food disagrees with you. You may like chocolate but know that it disagrees with you. That is not a dislike.

Acids: Arg n, *Bell*, China, Ign, Lyc, Nat m, Nux v, Ph ac, *Sulph*, Tub.

Alcoholic drinks: Ars, Bell, Calc, Cham, China, *Hyos*, Ign, Lyc, *Merc*, Nux v, Ph ac, Phos, Sil, Stram, Sulph.

Code: *TOP*, KEY, *Common*, Indicated

Alcoholic drinks, ale: NUX V

Alcoholic drinks, beer: BELL, Calc, *Cham*, CHINA, Med, Merc, Nat m, NUX V, Ph ac, *Phos*, Puls, Sep, *Sulph*.

Alcoholic drinks, whisky: Ign, *Merc*, Ph ac, Stram.

Alcoholic drinks, wine: ACON, *Carc*, *Ign*, LACH, *Merc*, Nat m, Nux v, Ph ac, Puls, Sil, *Sulph*, Tub.

Beans and peas: *Lyc*, Med, Nat m.

Bread: Calc, *CHINA*, Ign, KALI C, *Lyc*, NAT M, *Nit ac*, *Nux v*, *Ph ac*, *Phos*, PULS, *Sep*, SULPH, Tarant.

Bread, during pregnancy: *Sep*.

Breakfast: Lyc.

Butter: Ars, Carc, CHINA, *Merc*, *Nat m*, *Phos*, PULS.

Cabbage: Kali c, Lyc.

Cheese: *Arg n*, China, Nat m, *Nit ac*, *Sil*, *Staph*, Tub.

Cheese, strong: *Merc*, Nit ac, *Sulph*.

Coffee: *Acon*, *Bell*, CALC, Carc, *Caust*, *Cham*, *China*, *Lyc*, *Merc*, *Nat m*, NUX V, Ph ac, *Phos*, Puls.

Coffee, smell of: Lach, *Nat m*, Tub.

Drinks, cold: Acon, Ars, Lyc, Med, Nux v, Phos.

Drinks, warm: Caust, *Cham*, Med, PHOS, *Puls*.

Eggs: Bell, *Calc*, Carc, Nit ac, Phos, Puls, SULPH, Tub.

Farinaceous food, pasta etc.: Ars, Nat m, Phos.

Fats and rich food: *Ars*, *Bell*, *Calc*, *Carc*, CHINA, Lyc, *Merc*, NAT M, Nit ac, Phos, PULS, *Sep*, *Sulph*, Tarant.

Fish: Nat m, *Phos*, Sulph.

Fruit: ARS, Bar c, Bell, *Carc*, *Caust*, CHINA, Ign, Nat m, Phos, PULS.

Garlic: *Phos*.

Honey: *Nat m*.

***Meat:** *Arn*, *Ars*, *Aur*, CALC, Carc, CHINA, *Ign*, *Kali c*, *Lyc*, *Merc*, *Nat m*, *Nit ac*, NUX V, *Phos*, *Plat*, PULS, SEP, SIL, SULPH, *Tarant*, *Tub*.

Meat, beef: Merc.

Meat, fresh: *Thuja*.

Melons: *Ars*, *China*.

Code: *TOP*, KEY, *Common*, Indicated

Milk: *Arn, Ars, Calc, Carc,* IGN, *Phos, Puls,* Sep, Sil, STAPH, Sulph.

Milk, mother's: *Calc,* Lach, *Merc,* Nat m, SIL, Stram.

Olives: SULPH.

Oysters: Acon, Calc, Lyc, Med, *Phos,* Sep.

Pastry: *Ars,* Lyc, *Phos, Puls.*

Peas: Med.

Potatoes: *Phos,* Sep, Thuja.

Puddings: Ars, Calc, *Phos.*

Salt, salty food: *Carc,* China, Lyc, *Merc, Nat m,* Nit ac, Phos, Puls, *Sep,* Sil.

Slimy food: *Calc,* Med, *Nat m.*

Solid food: Bell, Lyc, Merc, *Staph,* Sulph.

Soup: *Arn,* Ars, Bell, Carc, Cham, China, Kali c, Lyc, Nat m, Puls, Staph.

Sour food: *Bell,* China, Ign, Lyc, Nat m, Nux v, Ph ac, *Sulph.*

Strawberries: China, *Sulph.*

Sugar: Ars, Caust, Merc, Phos.

Sweets (not the same as chocolate): *Arg n, Ars,* Bar c, Carc, CAUST, *Kali c, Lyc, Merc,* Nit ac, Nux v, *Phos,* Puls, *Sulph.*

Tea: *China,* Nux v, *Phos, Thuja.*

Tomatoes: *Phos.*

Turnips: Puls, Sulph.

Vegetables: Bell, Caust, *Nat m, Phos,* Sulph, Tub.

Water, cold: *BELL,* Caust, China, Nat m, NUX V, Phos, Puls, STRAM, Sulph.

PHYSICAL SHAPE INDEX

*Overweight: *Acon, Ars, Aur, Bell, CALC, Hyos, Kali c, Lyc, Phos, Puls, Sulph.*

Overweight, children: Bar c, Bell, *CALC.*

Stooped, round-shouldered: *Arg n, Aur, Calc,* Coloc, *Lyc,* Med, Nat m, Nux v, PHOS, *Sil,* SULPH, *Tub.*

Code: *TOP,* KEY, *Common,* Indicated

Thin: *Arg n*, Ars, Bar c, *Calc*, Caust, Ign, Lach, *Lyc*, Merc, Nat m, *Nit ac*, *Nux v*, Ph ac, *Phos*, Sep, *Sil*, SULPH, Tub.

SLEEP POSITION INDEX

This should only be considered if the person definitely takes up one position or knows that they have one posture which they prefer, even if at times they sleep in other positions. For example, Medorrhinum types say that they feel best sleeping on their fronts. It can also be useful when the person says, 'When I am upset I always sleep on my . . . .'

Back: Acon, Arn, Ars, Aur, *Calc*, Cham, China, Coloc, *Ign*, *Lyc*, Med, Nat m, Nit ac, *Nux v*, *Phos*, *Plat*, PULS, *Stram*, *Sulph*.

Back, hands on tummy: PULS.

Back, hands over head: Ars, Carc, Med, Nux v, Plat, PULS, Sulph.

Changed frequently: ARS, Aur, *Ign*, Kali c, Lach, Lyc, Phos, Plat.

Curled up, limbs drawn up: Anac, *Cham*, China, MERC, Nat m, *Plat*, PULS, *Stram*.

Feet out of the covers to cool them: Calc, CHAM, LACH, MED, *Phos*, *Plat*, PULS, *Sep*, Sil, SULPH.

Front: Ars, *Bell*, Calc, *Carc*, Caust, *Coloc*, Ign, Lach, *Lyc*, MED, *Nat m*, *Phos*, PULS, *Sep*, *Stram*, *Sulph*, *Tub*.

Head buried in pillow: Arn, Bell, Lach.

Head inclined backwards: *Bell*, China, Hyos, Ign, *Nux v*, Sep.

Head inclined forwards: Acon, Phos, Puls, Staph.

Head low: Arn, *Nux v*, Sil, Sulph.

Knees, on, face forced into pillow: *Carc*, *Lyc*, MED, *Phos*, *Sep*, *Tub*.

Knees and elbows, on: Calc, Carc, Lyc, *Med*, Phos, Sep, Stram, Tub.

Left side, on: Acon, Bar c, Calc, Carc, China, Merc, Nat m, Phos, Sep, *Sulph*.

Limbs spread apart: Bell, *Cham*, Nux v, Plat, *Puls*, Sulph.

Limbs stretched out: Bell, Cham, China, Plat, *Puls*.

Right side, on: *Ars*, Cham, China, Ign, Kali c, LACH, *Lyc*, Merc, PHOS, Sulph.

Code: *TOP*, KEY, *Common*, Indicated

UNUSUAL BODY SIGNS AND SYMPTOMS INDEX

Unusual signs and symptoms, or keynotes, are very useful in choosing remedies. Common symptoms are, in fact, the same for everyone, and consequently are not a useful indicator in finding a remedy, whereas unusual symptoms often are.

The list goes through the body area by area, starting at the top and working downwards. It is *not* complete; it is only a selection of interesting symptoms, missing out those that are common. The complete version runs to over one thousand closely typed pages! It is called *Kent's Repertory* and is available from the book suppliers listed in the appendix.

UNUSUAL SYMPTOMS AFFECTING THE WHOLE PERSON

*Autumn aggravates: *Calc, China, Coloc,* LACH, LYC, *Merc, Stram.*

Change of position ameliorates: Arn, Ars, Caust, *Cham*, IGN, Lach, Lys, *Ph ac*, Phos, Plat, *PULS*, Sep, Staph, Thuja.

Change of symptoms, constant: Carc, *Ign*, Kali c, *Puls, Tub.*

Clear weather aggravates: Acon, *Caust, Nux v.*

Cloudy weather ameliorates: *Caust.*

*Contradictory and alternating states: *Carc*, IGN, *Lyc, Nat m, Plat,* PULS, Sep, *Staph, Thuja*, TUB.

Dwarfish, small, undeveloped: BAR C, *Calc*, Carc, *Med, Sil, SULPH, Tub.*

*11 a.m. aggravates: *Nat m*, Nux v, Phos, Sep, SULPH.

Evening ameliorates: Arn, AUR, Carc, Lyc, MED, Nat m, Nux v, Puls, Sep.

Exercise ameliorates: *Arg n*, Calc, Carc, Caust, *Ign*, Kali c, Nat m, *SEP*, Sil, *TUB.*

*Faintness, fainting during periods: *Acon*, Calc, *Ign*, LACH, NUX V, *Puls*, SEP.

Faintness, fainting during pregnancy: *Bell, Kali c, Nux v, Puls, Sep.*

4 p.m.–6 p.m. aggravates: *Sep.*

*4 p.m.–8 p.m. aggravates: Coloc, *LYC*, Med, Sulph.

Code: *TOP*, KEY, *Common*, Indicated

---

*Heat, flushes of, with perspiration: CHINA, *Ign*, LACH, SEP, SULPH, TUB.

*Heat, flushes upwards: *Calc*, *Kali c*, *Lyc*, *Phos*, SEP, *Sulph*.

Morning ameliorates: LYC.

*Room full of people aggravates: *Arg n*, *Lyc*, *Phos*, *Puls*, *Sep*, *Sulph*.

Running ameliorates: Ars, Caust, *Ign*, Nat m, Nit ac, SEP, Sil, Tarant.

*Seashore aggravates: *Ars*, *Carc*, Med, *Nat m*, *Sep*, *Tub*.

Seashore ameliorates: Acon, *Carc*, *Hyos*, Lyc, *MED*, *Nat m*, Plat, Sep, Sil, *Stram*, *Tub*.

*Spring aggravates: *Aur*, BELL, CALC, LACH, LYC, *Nat m*, *Puls*, *Sep*, *Sil*, *SULPH*.

*Summer aggravates: BELL, LACH, *Lyc*, *Nat m*, *Nux v*, *Ph ac*, *Phos*, PULS.

Twilight aggravates: Arg n, *Ars*, *Calc*, *Caust*, Cham, Nat m, *Phos*, Plat, PULS, Staph.

Wet weather ameliorates: *Acon*, *Ars*, *Bell*, CAUST, Cham, MED, *Nit ac*, NUX V, *Plat*, *Sep*, *Sil*, Staph, Sulph.

*Winter aggravates: ACON, ARS, AUR, *Bar c*, *Bell*, *Calc*, *Caust*, *Cham*, *Hyos*, *Ign*, KALI C, LYC, *Merc*, NUX V, *Phos*, PULS, *Sep*, *Sil*, *Sulph*.

UNUSUAL SYMPTOMS OF VERTIGO AND GIDDINESS

Alcoholic drinks, from: COLOC, NAT M, *NUX V*.

Back, symptoms come up: SIL.

Body fluids, loss of: *China*, PHOS, Sep.

Closing eyes ameliorates: *Acon*, Lach, Puls, Sep, Sulph.

Coffee, after: *Arg n*, CHAM, NAT M, NUX V, Phos.

Dark room, entering: *Arg n*, *Stram*.

High places: ARG N, Aur, CALC, *Nat m*, Phos, Puls, Staph, SULPH.

Kneeling: SEP, Stram.

Lifting a weight: PULS.

Lying down: *Bell*, Caust, Nit ac, Nux v, Puls.

Code: *TOP*, KEY, *Common*, Indicated

Lying on right side aggravates: *Phos*, Tub.

Lying on left side aggravates: *Phos*, Sil.

Objects seem to be too far off: Anac, PULS, Stram.

Objects seem to turn in a circle, room whirls: *Calc*, CAUST, Merc, *NUX V, Phos*.

Old people, in: *Arn*, *Aur*, *Bar c*, *Phos*, Sulph.

Overuse of eyes: NAT M, PHOS, *Sil*.

Pregnancy, during: *Ars*, Bell, NAT M, Nux v, Phos.

Stairs, descending: Merc, *Plat*, Tarant.

Turning, in bed: BELL, Phos, Sulph.

Turning, on moving the head quickly: Bar c, CALC, *Coloc*, *Kali c*, Merc, PHOS, *Staph*, Sulph.

Walking in open air with sensation of gliding in the air: *China*, Hyos, Nat m, Sep, Stram, *Thuja*.

UNUSUAL SYMPTOMS OF THE HEAD

*Baldness: *Anac*, Arn, Aur, BAR C, Lyc, Med, Nat m, *Phos*, *Sep*, *Sil*, Sulph.

Baldness, in young people: *Bar c*, *Sil*, Tub.

Baldness, in patches: *Ars*, *Calc*, Lyc, *Phos*, Sep.

Beats against the bed: Ars, Hyos, Stram, Tarant, *Tub*.

Buries head in pillow: *Arn*, BELL, Lech, *Med*, *Stram*, Sulph, Tarant, TUB.

Cold air, sensitive to: *Ars*, *Bar c*, *Bell*, CHINA, Hyos, *Kali c*, *Lach*, *Lyc*, *Merc*, *Nat m*, NUX V, *Phos*, *Sep*, SIL, Thuja.

Dandruff, white: Ars, NAT M, *Phos*, THUJA.

Fontenelles, open (babies' skull bones that don't join up fast enough): CALC, *Merc*, Ph ac, *PHOS*, *Puls*, *Sep*, SIL, *Sulph*, Tub.

*Hair, dryness: *Calc*, *Kali c*, *Med*, *Phos*, *Sulph*, THUJA.

Hair, falling after giving birth: *Calc*, LYC, *Nat m*, *Nit ac*, *Sep*, Sil, SULPH.

Hair, falling during pregnancy: LACH.

*Hair, falling in spots: *Ars*, *Calc*, Nat m, *Phos*.

Hair, falling in handfuls: Lyc, PHOS, Sulph.

Code: *TOP*, KEY, *Common*, Indicated

Hair, goes grey: *Ars*, LYC, *Nat m*, *Ph ac*, *Sil*, *Staph*, *Sulph*, Thuja.
Hair, red: Lach, PHOS, SEP, Sulph.
Hair, tangles easily: Ars, Lyc, *Med*, Nat m, *Ph ac*, Sep, Sulph, Tub.
Hair, lustreless: Calc, *Med*, *Thuja*, Tub.
Heat, with coldness of extremities: *Arn*, Aur, BELL, *Calc*, Cann i, China, Lach, Lyc, Stram, Sulph.
Perspiration of scalp during sleep: *CALC*, *Cham*, *China*, *Lyc*, *Merc*, Nat m, *Sep*, *Sil*, Tub.
Tired feeling: Arn, Lach, Nat m, *PHOS*, Sil.

UNUSUAL SYMPTOMS OF HEADACHE

Cry out, pains compel one to: Anac, *Ars*, *Coloc*, Kali c, *Sep*, Sil, Stram, Tarant.
Cutting hair, after: BELL, Puls, *Sep*.
*Exertion of body, after: CALC, NAT M, *Nux v*.
Fasting, from: Ars, Caust, KALI C, Lach, *Lyc*, Nux v, *Phos*, *Sil*, *Sulph*, Thuja.
Fasting, from: if hunger is not appeased at once, must eat: *Lyc*, *Sulph*.
Forehead, middle, frontal sinuses from chronic coryza: *Ars*, SIL, *Thuja*.
*Hammering: *Ars*, BELL, *China*, *Lach*, NAT M, Sil, SULPH, *Tarant*.
Schoolgirls, in: Acon, Bell, *Calc*, NAT M, *PH AC*, *Phos*, Puls, *Sulph*, *Tub*.
Thunderstorms, before: Carc, Lach, PHOS, *Sep*, *Sil*.
Wind, cold, in: *Acon*, *Aur*, *Ign*, NUX V, *Sep*.

UNUSUAL SYMPTOMS OF THE EYES

Hair, sensation of, in the eye: PULS, Sil, Tarant.
*Hard lumps in the lids: Calc, *Sil*, SEP, STAPH, *Thuja*.
Inflammation, recurrent: *Ars*, CALC, *Sulph*.

Code: *TOP*, KEY, *Common*, Indicated

Opacity of cornea, arcus senilis: Acon, *Ars*, Calc, *Coloc*, Kali c, *Lyc*, *Merc*, Phos, PULS, *SULPH*.

Opening, difficulty in morning: Bar c, *Caust*, *Lyc*, *Nit ac*, *Ph ac*, *Sep*.

*Redness of edges: *Arg n*, ARS, *Coloc*, *Med*, *Nat m*, *Ph ac*, *Puls*, *SULPH*.

Styes, recurrent: Carc, Puls, *Sil*, Staph, SULPH, Tub.

Styes, inner corners: Bar c, *Nat m*, Sulph.

Watering, in cold air: Lyc, Phos, PULS, *Sep*, *Sil*, Sulph, Thuja.

UNUSUAL SYMPTOMS OF THE VISION

Blurred, before headache: Hyos, *Sep*, *Sulph*.

Dim, before headache: Hyos, Lach, *Nat m*, *Phos*, *Sep*, Sil, Stram, *Sulph*, *Tub*.

Feathery: *Calc*, LYC, *Merc*, Nat m.

Fiery, zigzags: Ign, NAT M, *Sep*.

Flashes in the dark: Arg n, PHOS, Stram.

Flickering, during headache: CHINA, *Coloc*, NAT M, *Phos*, *Sil*, *Sulph*.

Half sight, horizontal: ARS, *Aur*, *Lyc*, Sep, Sulph, *Tub*.

Half sight, lower lost: *Aur*, Sulph.

Half sight, upper lost: *Ars*, AUR.

Half sight, vertical: Aur, Calc, *Caust*, *Lyc*, *Nat m*, Sil.

UNUSUAL SYMPTOMS OF THE EARS

Discharges, purulent, with eczema: *Calc*, *Lyc*, *Merc*, *Sulph*.

Eruptions, cracks behind ears: *Lyc*, *Sep*, *Sulph*.

Fingers boring into ears, in child: *Sil*.

Frozen, as if: Caust, *PULS*.

Hearing, impaired for human voice: *Ars*, Calc, Ign, *PHOS*, *Sil*, *SULPH*.

Noises, synchronous with pulse: Ars, Coloc, Med, Merc, Nux v, Puls, Sep, Sil.

Code: *TOP*, KEY, *Common*, Indicated

Noises, reverberating: *Bar c*, Bell, *CAUST*, Kali c, *Lach*, LYC, Med, Merc, *Nit ac*, *Nux v*, *Ph ac*, *PHOS*, Plat, *Puls*, SEP, Sil, Sulph.

Pain, in cold air: *Ars*, *Cham*, Lach, *Lyc*, Merc, *Sep*.

Wax, increased: Bell, *Calc*, CAUST, Kali c, LACH, Lyc, Merc, Sep, Sil, Sulph, Tarant, Thuja.

UNUSUAL SYMPTOMS OF THE NOSE

Bleeding: see Epistaxis.

Discharge, burning skin, at night: NIT AC.

Discharge, scabs inside, green masses: *Phos*, SEP.

Discharge, scabs inside, hard to detach and leave it raw and sore: *Ars*, Nit ac, *Phos*, *Thuja*.

Discharge, scabs inside on septum (middle part): Anac, *Sil*, THUJA.

Epistaxis at menopause: Arg n, Bell, LACH, Nux v, Puls, Sep, *Sulph*.

Fingers, boring into nose: Anac, Arg n, Aur, Caust, Lyc, Merc, *Nat m*, *Ph ac*, Phos, SIL, Sulph, Tarant, Thuja.

Obstruction, open air ameliorates: Arg n, Kali c, *Phos*, *Sulph*.

Obstruction, in warm room: Arg n, Kali c, Phos, Plat, PULS, *Sulph*, Thuja.

Smell, acute, sensitive to odour of tobacco: *Bell*, China, *Ign*, *Nux v*, Phos, *Puls*.

Smell, acute, sensitive to unpleasant odours: *Acon*, Phos, SULPH.

Snuffles in new-born infants: LYC, *Merc*, NUX V, *Puls*.

UNUSUAL SYMPTOMS OF THE FACE

Discoloration, one side red, other pale: Acon, CHAM, *Lach*, *Nux v*, *Puls*, Sulph.

*Eruptions, cold sores around mouth: Ars, Med, NAT M, *Sep*.

Expression, fierce: *BELL*.

Expression, foolish: Arg n, *Bar c*, *Lyc*, *Phos*, *Stram*.

Expression, sleepy: CANN I, Phos.

Forehead, wrinkled chest symptoms: LYC.

Code: *TOP*, KEY, *Common*, Indicated

---

*Freckles: *Calc*, *Kali c*, LYC, *Nit ac*, PHOS, *Puls*, *Sep*, SULPH.

*Greasy: *Bar c*, *China*, Med, *Merc*, NAT M, *Tub*.

Lips, cracked, middle of lower lip: Calc, *Cham*, China, NAT M, Nux v, Ph ac, Phos, *Puls*, Sep.

Lips, cracked, middle of upper lip: *NAT M*.

Lips, numb: *Acon*, Calc, Caust, Lyc, *Nat m*, Phos, *Plat*.

Paralysis, one-sided: *Bar c*, *CAUST*, Puls, Sil.

Warts, on chin: *Lyc*, THUJA.

UNUSUAL SYMPTOMS OF THE MOUTH

Cheek, biting when talking or chewing: Anac, CAUST, Hyos, *IGN*, NIT AC.

Fingers, children putting in the mouth: *Calc*, *Cham*, Lyc, Med, Merc, Nat m, *Sil*, Tarant.

Gums bleed when cleaning teeth: Anac *Lyc*, Ph ac, Sep, *Staph*.

Odour, offensive in the morning: *Arg n*, AUR, Bell, Hyos, Lyc, Med, *Nux v*, PULS, *Sil*, Staph, Tub.

Open, during sleep: CALC, Caust, Cham, Ign, *Lyc*, Merc, *Nux v*, STRAM.

Speech, stammering (long exertion before one can utter a word, with distortion of face): STRAM.

Taste, bitter on waking in morning: SULPH.

Tongue, feels too broad: NAT M, PULS.

*Tongue, indented: ARS, Calc, MERC, *Puls, Sep*.

Tongue, one-sided numbness of: *Nat m*, Nux v.

UNUSUAL SYMPTOMS OF THE TEETH

Abscess of roots: *Bar c*, Calc, Caust, Lach, *Lyc*, *Merc*, SIL.

Decayed, hollow, premature in children: *Calc*, STAPH.

Decayed, hollow at roots: *Merc*, Sil, THUJA.

Grinding during sleep: Acon, ARS, BELL, CANN I, *Hyos*, Ign, *Kali c*, Merc, *Stram*, *Sulph*, TUB.

Pain, toothache after filling: ARN, Merc, NUX V, Sep, Staph.

Code: *TOP*, KEY, *Common*, Indicated

*Teething, difficult: ACON, *Arn*, ARS, *Bell*, CALC, *CHAM*, *Ign*, *Lyc*, MERC, SIL, STAPH, SULPH.

Teething, slow: *Calc*, SIL, *Sulph*, Thuja, TUB.

Wisdom teeth, ailments from eruption of: *Calc*, *Cham*, *Sil*.

UNUSUAL SYMPTOMS OF THE THROAT

Adenoids: Bar c, Calc, Merc, Sulph, *Thuja*, Tub.

*Choking, constriction while drinking: HYOS, *NAT M*.

Choking, constriction while eating: Anac, *Kali c*, LACH, Nit ac.

Pain, in damp weather: CALC, Lach.

Pain, from warmth and warm drinks: Carc, LACH, *Lyc*, Merc.

Pain, warm drinks and warmth ameliorate: ARS, *Cham*, LYC, Nux v, *Sulph*.

Tonsils, hard: BAR C, Calc, *Cham*, *Ign*, *Nit ac*, Sil, *Staph*, Thuja.

UNUSUAL SYMPTOMS OF THE NECK

Clothing aggravates: Arg n, *Bell*, Carc, Caust, *Kali c*, *LACH*, Merc, Nux v, *Sep*, Sulph, *Tarant*, Tub.

Glands, hardening like knotted cords: Bar c, Calc, Lyc, *Merc*, Nit ac, *Sil*, *Sulph*, TUB.

Goitre left: *Lach*.

Goitre right: Ars, Caust, Kali c, *Lyc*, Nit ac, *Phos*, *Sep*, Sil.

Redness, in spots: BELL, Nux v, Sep, Tarant.

Torticollis, drawn to left: *Bell*, Lyc, *Nux v*, PHOS.

Torticollis, drawn to right: Caust, *Lyc*.

UNUSUAL SYMPTOMS OF THE STOMACH

Note: the stomach is just below the ribs and mainly on the left-hand side and in the middle. It is not the same as the abdomen.

*Appetite, increased at night: CHINA, *Ign*, LYC, PHOS.

Code: *TOP*, KEY, *Common*, Indicated

*Appetite, ravenous with wasting away: Bar c, CALC, China, Lyc, NAT M, *Phos*, *Sulph*, *Tub*.

*Appetite, lack of with thirst instead: *Calc*, *Phos*, SULPH.

Disordered, after bread: CAUST, Lyc, *Merc*, Nat m, Nit ac, Puls, *Sep*.

Disordered, after fat food: *Caust*, PULS, *Sep*, *Sulph*.

Disordered, after fruit: ARS, CHINA, Lyc.

Disordered, after ice cream: ARS, PULS.

Disordered, after oysters: LYC.

Disordered, after vexation: CHAM.

Distension, eructations ameliorate: Arg n, Carc.

Distension, eructations do not ameliorate: *China*, *Lyc*, Phos.

Emptiness, weak feeling around 11 a.m.: *Phos*, *SULPH*.

Pain, after excitement: CHAM, COLOC, Nux v, *Staph*.

Pain, after vexation: Acon, Ars, Cham, Ign, Phos, STAPH.

Seasickness: Nat m, NUX V, *Sep*, *Staph*.

Travel sickness: *Calc*, Carc, *Lyc*, Nat m, *Nux v*, Phos, Puls, SEP, Sulph.

Ulcers: Arg n, *Ars*, *Bell*, *Kali c*, *Lach*, LYC, *Merc*, *Nit ac*, *Nux v*, PHOS, SEP.

Vomiting, after anger: CHAM, COLOC, NUX V, Staph.

Vomiting, after drinking a very small amount: ARS, PHOS.

Vomiting, as soon as liquid becomes warm in stomach: PHOS.

Vomiting, before periods: *Calc*, Cham, China, *Nux v*, *Puls*, Sulph.

Vomiting bile in the morning: *SEP*, Tarant.

Vomiting, immediately after drinking: ARS, *Nux v*.

Vomiting, immediately after eating: ARS, CALC, Hyos, LACH, NUX V, PHOS, PULS.

Vomiting mucus from cough: *Nit ac*, *Puls*, *Sil*, Thuja, Tub.

Vomiting, when putting hands in warm water: *Phos*.

UNUSUAL SYMPTOMS OF THE ABDOMEN

This is the area from about two inches below the ribs down to the pubic line. It is not the stomach.

Code: *TOP*, KEY, *Common*, Indicated

---

*Clothing, sensitive to: ARG N, CALC, *Caust*, *China*, LACH, LYC, NUX V, *Sep*.

Distension, in children: ARG N, BAR C, CALC, CAUST, *Lyc*, *SIL*, *SULPH*.

Eruptions, shingles: Ars, Merc, Sulph, Thuja.

Falling out, sensation of: Coloc, Kali c, Nat m, *Nux v*, SEP.

Impaction: BELL, Caust, Lach.

Haemorrhoids, pain from: Coloc, Lach, NUX V, Puls, *Sulph*.

Live object, sensation of in abdomen: *THUJA*.

Pain, aching, bending double ameliorates: *Bell*, Carc, *Caust*, *China*, COLOC, KALI C, *Lach*, PULS.

Pain, aching, dull flexing limbs ameliorates: *Bell*, COLOC, *Sep*.

Pain, at period, ameliorated flow becomes free: Bell, Kali c, LACH, Sep, Sulph.

Pain, bearing down in periods: SEP.

Pain, like sharp stones rubbing together: COLOC, Staph.

Pain, liver extending to back: *Kali c*, LYC, *Nat m*.

Pendulous abdomen: Aur, Bell, Plat, SEP.

UNUSUAL SYMPTOMS OF THE RECTUM

Diarrhoea, at 5am: *Phos*, SULPH, Tub.

Diarrhoea, after anticipation: *Arg n*, *Ph ac*.

Diarrhoea, after beer: China, Lyc, SULPH.

Diarrhoea, before periods: LACH, Phos, *Sil*, Tub.

*Diarrhoea, on waking, with urgency: SULPH.

*Stool, incomplete evacuation of: LYC, Nat m, Nit ac, NUX V, *Sep*, *Sulph*.

UNUSUAL SYMPTOMS OF THE BLADDER

Bedwetting in first sleep: *CAUST*, *Ph ac*, Phos, Puls, *SEP*, Tub.

Paralysis, no desire after giving birth: ARS, *CAUST*, *Hyos*, Nux v, Phos.

Code: *TOP*, KEY, *Common*, Indicated

Polypi: Ars, CALC, Lyc, Merc, Phos, Puls, Sil, Staph, Thuja.

Urging to constantly urinate during prolapses of uterus: *SEP.*

Urging to urinate during pregnancy: Acon, *Puls*, Sulph.

*****Urination, involuntary during cough:** *Bell*, CALC, *CAUST*, Kali c, *Lyc*, *NAT M*, *Nux v*, Ph ac, *Sep*.

Urination, involuntary from laughing: *CAUST*, *Nat m*, *Nux v*, *Puls*, *SEP*, Tarant.

Urination, involuntary if desire is resisted: Calc, Merc, Nat m, *Puls*, Sep, *Sulph*, *Thuja*.

Urination, involuntary when blowing nose: CAUST, Nat m, Puls.

UNUSUAL SYMPTOMS OF THE MALE GENITALS

Masturbation, in children: *Bar c*, *Carc*, Hyos, *Med*, Ph ac, Plat, Staph, Tub.

Penis, atrophy of: *Arg n*, *Cann i*, IGN, LYC, Staph.

Sex, aversion to: Caust, Kali c, Lach, *LYC*, Nat m, Phos, Staph.

Swelling of testicles from mumps: *PULS.*

Testicles, atrophy of: *Arg n*, *Aur*, Bar c, Staph.

UNUSUAL SYMPTOMS OF FEMALE GENITALS

*****Hair, falling out:** *NAT M*, *Nit ac*.

Insensibility, of vagina: *Phos*, SEP.

Itching, during pregnancy: Calc, *Merc*, *SEP*.

*****Sex, aversion to:** CAUST, *Lyc*, *Med*, NAT M, *Phos*, *SEP*, *Sulph*.

Thrush, gushing: CALC, LYC, SEP, SIL, Thuja.

Thrush, at puberty: SEP.

Vagina, dryness of: *Acon*, *Ars*, *Bell*, *Lyc*, *NAT M*, Puls, *Sep*, Tarant.

*****Vagina, pain in during sex:** ARG N, Kali c, *NAT M, Plat, SEP*, Staph, Sulph, Thuja.

Code: *TOP*, KEY, *Common*, Indicated

UNUSUAL SYMPTOMS OF BREATHING

Asthmatic, after midnight: ARS, *Lach*.
Asthmatic, after midnight, must spring out of bed: ARS.
Asthmatic, 2 a.m.: ARS, Med.
Asthmatic, 2 a.m.–3 a.m.: KALI C.
Asthmatic, 2 a.m.–4 a.m.: Med.
Asthmatic, 3 a.m.: CHINA, KALI C.
*Asthmatic, children: *Acon*, Ars, Bell, *CALC*, CHAM, *Ign*, PULS.
*Asthmatic, old people: ARS, *Bar c*.
Rattling, in old people: *Bar c*, LYC.

UNUSUAL SYMPTOMS OF COUGHING

Chest, must hold with both hands while coughing: ARN, Merc, Nat m, *Phos*, *Sep*.
Cough, going from warm to cold and vice versa: Acon, Carc, Caust, Cham, Lach, Merc, Nux v, PHOS, Sep.
Head, must hold with both hands while coughing: *NUX V*, Sulph.
Larynx, touching lightly aggravates: Bell, China, *LACH*, Staph, Stram.
Sit up, must: *Ars*, Caust, Hyos, Lach, *PHOS*, *PULS*, *Sep*, Staph.
Sleep, preventing: Anac, Bell, Caust, Kali c, LYC, Nux v, Phos, PULS, SEP, *Sulph*, Tub.
Teething during: Acon, Bell, Calc, *Cham*, Hyos.

UNUSUAL SYMPTOMS OF THE CHEST

Breast, atrophy of: Anac, Ars, Bar c, Lach, Nit ac.
Breastbone, pain in when coughing: *Ars*, *Caust*, *China*, Kali c, *Phos*, Sep, Sil, Staph, SULPH, Thuja.
Breasts, lumps in: Aur, Carc, Cham, China, Coloc, *Lyc*, *Nit ac*, *Phos*, Puls, SIL, *Sulph*, Tub.
Eruptions, boils under armpits, recurrent: Lyc.
Eruptions, shingles: LACH, Staph, Thuja.

Code: *TOP*, KEY, *Common*, Indicated

Heart, palpitation during digestion: LYC, *Sep.*

Heart, palpitation from frustration: Acon, Arg n, CHAM, *Ign*, *Nat m*, SEP, Staph.

Heart, palpitation on going to sleep: *Calc*, *Nat m*, Phos, Sil, SULPH.

Heart, palpitation while lying: *Ars*, Carc, *Lach*, Lyc, Merc, NAT M, NUX V, PULS, Sep, SULPH.

Heart, sensation of heart having stopped: *Arg n*, *Aur*, *Lach.*

Milk, in non-pregnant women: Ars, Bell, Calc, Lyc, *Merc*, Phos, PULS, Stram, *Tub.*

Milk, mother's, child refuses: *Calc*, Lach, *Merc*, Nat m, *Ph ac*, Sulph.

Nipples, retraction of: Carc, Lach, *Sil*, Tub.

Perspiration, offensive, from arm pits: Calc, *Lach*, *Lyc*, NIT AC, Sep, SIL, SULPH.

UNUSUAL SYMPTOMS OF THE BACK

Backache, compelled to walk bent: *Cann i*, *Kali c*, *Sep*, *Sulph.*

Backache, from prolonged stooping: *NAT M.*

Backache, lying on something hard ameliorates: Bell, *Kali c*, NAT M, Puls, *Sep.*

Dorsal spine, curvature of: Bar c, *Calc*, *Lyc*, Puls, Sil, Thuja.

Neck region, perspiration at night: CALC, SULPH, Tub.

Neck region, perspiration in sleep: CALC, *Lach*, Med, Ph ac, *Phos.*

Spine, curvature of with pain: LYC, SIL.

Straining, easily done: CALC, LYC, *Nux v*, Ph ac, *Sep.*

UNUSUAL SYMPTOMS OF THE ARMS AND LEGS

*Arthritic nodosities of finger joints: CALC, CAUST, *Lach*, LYC, *Med*, *Sil*, *Staph*, *Sulph.*

Arthritic nodosities of finger joints, with stiffness: LYC.

*Bursae: *ARN*, *NAT M*, SIL.

*Bunions on feet: *Phos*, SIL.

Code: *TOP*, KEY, *Common*, Indicated

Callosities, on soles: *Ars*, *Calc*, SIL.

Calves, cramps on stretching in bed: *CALC*, *Sulph*.

Chilblains, on toes: *Nit ac*, *Nux v*, *PULS*.

*Eruptions, in bends of joints: NAT M, *Sep*.

*Hands, restless must fidget: *Ars*, *Hyos*, *Sulph*, TARANT.

Knees, cold at night: *PHOS*, Sep.

Knees, pain in when descending steps: Kali c, Merc, Nit ac.

Pain, on beginning to move: *Caust*, Lach, LYC, *Med*, Nit ac, Ph ac, PHOS, PULS, *Sil*, Thuja, Tub.

*Stumbling, when walking: ARG N, BAR C, *Calc*, CAUST, *Hyos*, IGN, *Lach*, *Nat m*, *Ph ac*, *Phos*, Tub.

Toes, cracked skin between: *Lach*, *Nat m*, SIL.

Toes, cracked skin with violent itching: NAT M.

Warts, close to finger nails: *CAUST*, *Lyc*, Nat m, Sep.

UNUSUAL SYMPTOMS OF DREAMS

*Exertion, making great physical effort: ARS.

*Falling, from high places: *Sulph*, THUJA.

Falling, into water: Ign, Merc, Ph ac, Puls, Sep, Sulph.

Repeating: *Arg*, Ign, Nat m.

Snakes: Arg n, Carc, Kali c, Lach, Sep, Sil, Tub.

UNUSUAL SYMPTOMS OF SLEEP

Sleeplessness after 3 a.m.: ARS, *Calc*, *China*, *Nux v*, *SEP*, *SULPH*, *THUJA*, TUB.

Sleeplessness, after 4 a.m.: Caust, Lyc, Nit ac, Ph ac, Phos, Sep, Staph, *SULPH*, Thuja.

Sleeplessness, from grief: Carc, *Ign*, Lach, NAT M, *Sulph*.

Sleeplessness, from vexation: Acon, Ars, Calc, Cham, Coloc, Nux v, Staph.

Code: *TOP*, KEY, *Common*, Indicated

UNUSUAL SYMPTOMS OF THE SKIN

Eruptions, circular: *Bar c*, *Calc*, Carc, Med, *NAT M*, *Phos*, *SEP*, *Sulph*, *Thuja*, *TUB*.
Itching, wool aggravates: Phos, Puls, Sulph, Tub.
Urticaria, after violent exertion: Calc, *Nat m*.
White spots: *Aur*, *Calc*, *Merc*, *Phos*, *Sep*, SIL, *Sulph*.

COMMON CAREERS AND ACTIVITIES THAT INDICATE REMEDIES

This is really just a bit of lighthearted fun, but it also emphasizes that a person's choice of career is a potentially important indication of their deepest inner trauma.

Actors   Thuja
Aerobics enthusiasts   Tarantula, Sepia
Alexander teachers   Kali carb
Artists   Phosphorus, (very refined and delicate) China
Authors of many books   Lachesis
Business people   Nux vomica
Bosses   (argumentative) Kali carb, (dictatorial) Lycopodium, (ambitious and hard-working) Nux vomica
Churchwardens   Thuja
Collectors   Arsenicum
Collectors of junk   Sulphur
Criminals   Anacardium
Dancers   Sepia, Carcinosin, (fast, twitchy dancing) Tarantula
Diary keepers   Lachesis
Directors of professional bodies   Kali carb, Lycopodium
Evangelists   Argentum nitrate
Explorers   Tuberculinum
Helpers, true rescuers   Natrum mur
Inventors   Sulphur
Judges   Arsenicum, Lycopodium
Laughing people   Cannabis indica
Mafiosi   Thuja
Marathon runners   Natrum mur
Museum curators   Arsenicum, Sulphur

Code: *TOP*, KEY, *Common*, Indicated

Musicians (bagpipes) Lycopodium (windbags), (classical and leaders of orchestras) Aurum, (organists) Thuja, (conductors) Lycopodium, (solo singers) Platina.
Nudists Hyoscyamus
Nursery teachers Pulsatilla, Stramonium
Obstetricians Stramonium
Philosophers Sulphur
Police officers Anacardium, Lycopodium
Pop stars (pull loose their neck tie) Lachesis, Platina, (strip and act lewdly on stage) Hyoscyamus, Tarantula, Medorrhinum (mega-stars)
Pornographers Hyoscyamus
Professors Lycopodium
Prostitutes Medorrhinum
Psychics and mystics Phosphorus, Silica
Scriptwriters for soap operas Medorrhinum
Singers Lachesis
Students, long-term Silica
Swimmers Pulsatilla
Traffic wardens Lycopodium
Travel agents Tuberculinum
Vengeful neighbours Nitric acid
Vets Natrum mur
Victims, professional Staphisagria

CHAPTER NINE

Trauma Patterns

WHY PATTERNS?

Some researchers have delved into the memories of very old people who remember the childhood stories of their grandparents. By this means they reached back 200 years. They discovered that the same trauma themes were current then as now. Shakespeare and the Greek myths mention them too. The trauma patterns of our society have probably not changed for thousands of years. In fact they have probably always been the same and there are relatively few main patterns of suffering.

A person as a trauma pattern can be likened to a musical instrument and a musician – the soul seeking expression and experience through the instrument of the body.

Initially let us suppose that the person is a piano, in need of repair. The homoeopathic remedy first repairs the dampers and stuck keys and then retunes it. As the person becomes healthier perhaps they change the music to something more to their soul's liking and become more adept at playing. After a while, as their health improves more, they have the idea of composing their own music. Later still with increasing competence they become 'at one' with the instrument and the music it produces becomes transcendent: what is heard is only the music and the instrument fades away – soul-to-soul communication. But the person is still a piano. Generally people do not change from their early pattern; the original instrument is still the one they play, perhaps with minor variations – other keyboard instruments for example – but this is not restricting to their soul.

So in this model we are each a musical instrument, formed

in the early part of our life, and the homoeopathic task is to help the person make good use of it.

TRAUMA PATTERN DESCRIPTIONS

These are divided, sometimes rather artificially, into three sections: stresses, attitude (sometimes also keynotes) and likely diseases and illnesses.

Stress as a causation also relates to the particular vulnerability of the person. Either can be looked at as cause or effect since the pattern is as ancient as the human race, but homoeopaths favour the idea that the vulnerability is the problem that makes causes appear to be true. (If you are vulnerable to insults then you may notice them particularly and they will hurt you; if you are not, you are more likely to observe dispassionately that the other person offers insults.)

In considering which remedy to use, the stresses and trauma attitude (keynote) are the main criteria.

The trauma as disease section is intended only as a hint on common pathology and as an occasional guide. Under no circumstances should disease be used as the initial criterion for selecting a remedy. It is a helpful confirmation at best.

Not all the trauma patterns corresponding to remedies listed in the indexes are given. The most common ones are, but many rarely used ones are left out to keep the book as clear and useful as possible. Good references are given if you want to use a rarer remedy or delve deeper.

Each trauma pattern has its own core image and the remedies can treat the old and infirm as well as infants and children and healthy adults. So each trauma pattern has differing facets in differing age groups. For example, earache is common in children but uncommon in older people, so this must be borne in mind when reading the patterns as sometimes you have to stretch your imagination to see the remedy in a different age group.

There can be different 'faces' within the adult patterns; for example, the philosophical Sulphur and the practical Sulphur.

There is also a polarity or 'flip side' to each pattern; for example, people can exhibit the nice or the nasty aspect of the remedy. Lycopodium can be dictators but extremely lacking in confidence. Kali carb can be strong or feeble. Some patterns show both aspects operating at once, or the different sides coming into play in different situations; Lycopodium, for example can be dictators at home and submissive in the workplace or vice versa.

Each pattern has an inside and an outside facet. The inside state is often the softer, weaker, more vulnerable aspect which sometimes shows up as the real state in a young person. The outer state is usually a compensation for the inner state, the ego nature externalized, a defensive posture to protect the inner weakness. It is important to understand that everyone has an outer personality, a way of presenting to the world that is a front behind which their inner, more vulnerable, weaker, childlike, immature, unloved, 'stuck' person hides. Many of the world's problems are based on conflicts between these outer masks and the inner realities on a mass level. These protected postures are necessary compensations for survival in children growing up in a hostile or unloving world, but if we retain them as adults in caring relationships when they have outlived their usefulness they become prisons and defences against love, protecting us from the very things that we want. Homoeopathic remedies can be seen as softening and dissolving tools for these outer defences so that the love flows in.

We are all surrounded by many loving sources all our lives; but we have learnt to retreat to safe, closed off places which keep love out. For example, Arsenicum types are very critical. They criticize others openly or mentally and thus keep them at a distance. Who would want to be close to such a person? They also criticize their own behaviour and by putting themselves down, denigrate the inner person. So the remedy helps tone down the criticism level, letting other people feel warmer towards them and reducing the self-criticism, so that the inner person can feel the warmth and gain confidence and strength.

Sometimes the trauma pictures are too crude. For example, when you meet someone for the first time, your first impression may be of haughtiness or arrogance. This may be the only time you witness arrogance but believe it. However, if you are haughty yourself you will naturally find this characteristic in others as a reflection; so if everyone seems to have a similar aspect then it is probably not theirs. Self-awareness is essential to unprejudiced observation, a key quality in homoeopathy.

And these pictures or patterns also reflect my bias. They are difficult word pictures to paint and the artist is part of the process, so you have my choice of colourings, my blind spots, my wrinkles. There is a difficult balance between picture, bias and the many faces of people, so please be tolerant of the result and try to understand the fluid, multi-faceted image I am trying to project to you.

ACONITE

Keyword   **Shock**
Source   **Plant**

Stresses

Shock is the keyword. Fear and fright from shock are very strong here, the strongest fears of all the homoeopathic types. *Great panic and fear of death.* Great shock from seeing an accident or hearing about the sudden death of someone known to them *not* terror or sustained fear, which is more Stramonium.

Tremendous problems associated with fear and fright, bad news. Also anger with anxiety, fright and silent grieving. They can be upset by overexcitement and excessive joy. Humiliation and hurrying also upset them. A chill or a very cold dry wind, forms of sudden shock, can make them instantly ill.

Attitude

Vital, vigorous, extrovert, robust people who are yet exquisitely sensitive to mental shock, such as an earthquake, being trapped in a lift, lights going out in a tunnel, accidents, or a weaker person suffering from a big shock.

They act as if death is imminent; fear of death is very strong (but this may not be obvious; you have to try to get inside their mental state). Intense claustrophobia, even driving in a car on a motorway, as well as in lifts, etc. Great fear of earthquakes (another shock).

Sympathetic and friendly.

Trauma as disease

Claustrophobia. Strong phobias from any shock or fright, completely out of proportion to the event.

Sudden intense illnesses. Strong *panic* attacks especially if triggered by a similar event to the original shock. Palpitations.

ANACARDIUM

Keywords **Total isolation**
Source **Marking nut**

Stresses

Isolation and separation at birth or after, causing great loss of self-esteem. Being put down; they work hard under adverse conditions to prove themselves, then break down.

Violent repression, often justified as 'discipline'.

Attitude

Tremendous inferiority, lack of confidence reflected in cruelty, insensitivity and murderous aggressiveness. Violent fantasies. Image of the lone wolf, with bared teeth, yet lacking the confidence to attack.

A feeling of powerlessness. They must prove themselves, feeling that they are a nobody and wanting desperately to be loved and accepted.

Situations where the person's sense of self-esteem is very dependent on achievements, such as passing exams, getting promotion, etc. If they do not succeed, lack of confidence and conflict develop and separation and isolation appear.

Children may pull flies apart or draw wolves. Stalin drew wolves as his main doodle at meetings. These people can appear very timid at first. They always feel like outsiders, alone, without anyone there for them, however hard they try.

There is a sort of dual personality, either very nice or very nasty with not much in between.

The sequence of events as the criminal type grows up is something like this. The father beats the child harshly and cruelly; the mother condones this, or is perhaps also beaten, and the child becomes hard and unfeeling in response to the violence. At school the child be appreciated and channel their energy into study as this gains them approval and 'love'. But if they try too hard and fail, or are criticized, they rapidly lose confidence. They start to pick on others and tease them. Because of this behaviour, they begin to lose the sympathy of adults and become cut off from love and care. They start to bully and intimidate others and as this compounds the situation they become gang leaders, vicious and violent, and drift to crime.

In the broken or extreme state, Anacardiums are murderers or people who but for their self-control would be murderers: people associated with old age, death by design, euthanasia, soldiers who have killed in battle, dictators who murder and police attracted to murder are all potential candidates. So might be a vicious judge.

Keynotes

Lack of confidence, the lowest.
Duality, division, isolation, loneliness.
Enjoys cruelty, violence, swearing, great inferiority inside, feels better by eating. But they are often non-violent, just seeking approval.
Sensation of band round body parts ('psychological hand cuffs' or 'on a lead').
Cold hard look.

Trauma as disease

Crimes of violence and cruelty. Prisoners. Living in isolation. Schizophrenia. Cruel dictators.

ARGENTUM NITRATE

Keyword **Impulsive**
Source **Silver**

Stresses

Early separation with isolation and some form of time pressure, with panic if it is not achieved. Likely to be a separation after a hasty birth process, with some panic and rush. Anticipation.

Attitude

Impulsiveness and time pressure characterize these people*. They tend towards insensitivity because they do not give themselves time to feel. They act first and think second, saying things before thinking about them. They are extrovert, open, friendly, straightforward, even evangelical, and can like public speaking. They get sore throats from excessive speaking and singing.

Gullibility goes with this lack of thinking power and naivety of thought; for example having an affair without thinking about it and later confessing to the spouse.

Everything bursts out of them* – wind, burps, thoughts, stool by way of nervous diarrhoea. They often suffer from irritable bowel syndrome.

They are superstitious about cracks in paving stones, corners, etc. and have fears about what might have happened, imaginary events that flash through their minds.

They have strong fears of claustrophobia*, crossing bridges*, lifts, planes and being enclosed; also fear of high places because of the impulse to jump*.

They hurry and become anxious, and walk faster from the anxiety. They are very fearful of arriving late or early for an appointment*, or missing a deadline.

They have strong feelings of being alone and abandoned, even isolated*.

They are fearful too of doing things in case they do not get it right*.

Keynotes

Extremely nervous before important events*, especially public speaking which they like to do, impulsively letting their mind roll.

Very hot people, with some exceptions. Crave salt and sweets, yet sweet and sugary things can often upset their digestion.

Claustrophobia and agoraphobia (fear of closed and open spaces), fear of high places because they may jump.

Trauma as disease

Birth trauma. All the signs marked with an asterisk above could come from a birth experience, one where there is an enforced delivery, an induction perhaps, followed by rush and panic, and being abandoned directly after the birth, while perhaps the mother recovers from the excessive pain or the complications from having been rushed, etc.

Digestive disorders, with nervous diarrhoea typical especially after sugar. Wind, especially belching. Periodic weakness. Tremendous palpitations. Ulcers of the eye. Splinterlike pains.

ARNICA

Keyword **Bruised**
Source **Plant**

This is the main remedy for trauma which is primarily physical, with *bruising*, with or without a shock or emotional content. When it is purely shock think of Aconite, when terror Stramonium, but for pure injury (falling down shafts or stairs, being punched, going through windscreens or just banging the head) Arnica has no equal. It is a miracle in action. It should be in every medical kit in every home; it is a basic essential to life.

However, it has deeper uses. It is wonderful for symptoms like soreness from an old – even a twenty-year-old – injury.

This is because the trauma is just as alive now as when it happened. Arnica can easily reach back twenty or more years. It is also very good for things like repetitive injury from deformed joints such as the effects of polio. It can be very helpful for pains from unavoidable repeating injury.

ARSENICUM

Keyword   **Tidy**
Source   **Arsenic**

Stresses

A deep sense of anger arising from not being cared for when very young. In infancy they never felt secure and grew up trying to compensate for this. Probably received a lot of criticism as they grew up and not much caring.

Attitude

Arsenicum is for the obsessively tidy. They have immaculately tidy places to live in, everything in its place and very well ordered, and dress with the same sense, very smart, often with gold extras such as watches, jewellery, etc.

They come from an essentially selfish perspective, seeking security through ownership, of others (their husbands, wives, children), of money, of possessions, but especially of people. They control others through their money. They look upon things from a 'What's in it for me?' perspective. If their partner is ill their inner response is 'What will happen to me if they die?' and fear of death is very high on their fearful agenda.

All this tidiness and need to control comes out of a deep rage and insecurity, something from early childhood, a deep need to create a feeling of security through order and owning. They are not aware of this.

Arsenicum fears to be alone, wants company and worries excessively about their own health.

Initially Arsenicum is seen as having lots of colds, thirst for sips and chilliness, along with restlessness, after midnight being their worst time. The typical picture is of waking in the middle of the night and pacing up and down in an anguished, restless state saying that they are dying and that you must get the doctor, when often the complaint is quite minor. Later as they become more ill they develop more fear, especially fear of death, a tremendous anxiety about their health, which deep down is a fear of dying, and a great need for company.

Arsenicum often develops asthmalike symptoms after the excessive use of antibiotics given by the doctor under the pressure of the patient's anxiety and frequency of colds. Indeed, because of their insecurities, Arsenicums are the most likely people to suffer medical abuse of this type. They seek attention for every ailment and receive far too much controlling treatment, more than their constitution can bear. Fault-finding, criticism, anguish, despair of recovery and suicide can follow later on in life.

Psychodynamics

These are very angry people who are very critical of others and themselves. They often make malicious jokes which they think are funny but which the butt of the jokes feels are cruel; they do it automatically and do not realize that this is why they feel alone and insecure in a hostile world. They poison their environment. They can be so angry that they feel the impulse to kill others and when they turn this anger in on themselves they create guilt, sadness, despair, and eventually the desire to kill themselves. They try to kill themselves by hanging or unconsciously by asthma, Arsenicum's main pathology which, like hanging, is suffocation. They become sad when alone because there is no one on whom to take out their anger by malicious jokes. They are scared when alone because deep down they feel the impulse to kill themselves and this is also the reason for their fear of death.

Keynotes

Tidiness, restlessness, anxiety, wakefulness, fault-finding, fears of illness, death and robbers, meanness, greed, hoarding out of great inner insecurity.

Burning pains relieved by hot drinks or hot things are very characteristic. Burning discharges, red around the nostrils, are classic signs in colds.

Trauma as disease

Asthma. Worse at night, originally from colds that go direct to the chest after a period of using antibiotics.

AURUM

Keyword **Serious duty**
Source **Gold**

Stresses

Take offence easily, easily feel humiliated when criticized or told off, from contradiction or from argument.
Devastated by broken love affairs and tend to take revenge on the next lover.
Abandonment at birth, after birth, in the first years of life. An idealistic achiever with high goals.

Attitude

Aurum is a prime remedy for a deeply wounded heart and is one of the major suicide remedies. Aurums need not be the suicidal type, but many are. They are serious people who listen to classical music to relieve them of their painful feelings; it helps them process and live out their suppressed and desperately sad feelings.
Aurums can be very high achievers until things go wrong; they are serious, aloof, intimidating and arrogant with a strong drive to build a career, seeking achievement and praise, like the appreciation that gold receives. They can have a strong sense of duty and its counterpoint, guilt, and are fine while at or aiming for the top, but not when they start to fail.

And being very susceptible to criticism, they can fail easily if they are criticized or if their plan is frustrated in some way.

Such individuals may take refuge in addictive behaviours and drug or alcohol abuse as well as in religion and suicide.

As well as the intense idealistic student who starts to fail badly at school after being top of the class, Aurum can be the millionaire whose empire crashes into ruins.

Here is a direct quote from a newspaper story.

> 'We had no idea he was suicidal,' said the mother of a 24 year old man who hanged himself after his girlfriend was killed in a road accident. 'With hindsight we should have noticed he was deeply depressed. From being someone who's been extrovert suddenly he spent more time alone, listening to music and withdrawing from the world.'

This captures the image well.

Aurums under stress become reckless and will, for example, drive fast and into oncoming traffic. However, because guilt and its reflex, duty, run very high in this type, suicide is frequently a very strong desire which is not always acted out. Instead they may seek salvation in religion, in meditation practice and spiritual activities which they take very seriously, or in another strong 'dutiful' profession or activity as a reflex to their suicidal thoughts and their sense of worthlessness. So frequently they are regular church goers, meditators or ashram devotees, even long after the 'guru' has died. Or they become very responsible people, achieving great positions in life, perhaps in religious activities.

They often feel better in the evenings.

Keynotes

Dutiful, guilty, serious, high achievers, cannot take criticism, better for classical music, religious, serious meditators, intimidating.

Traumas as disease

Depression and suicidal inclinations, joyless in the extreme. With suppression of anger, fear and other feelings they develop angina and heart circulatory symptoms. Often testicular problems, especially the right one.

All pains worse at night. Heart problems. Tremendously painful headache, boring over the right eye.

BARYTA CARBONICUM

Keyword **Backward**
Source **Carbonate of barium**

Stresses

Anticipation. Small events.

Attitude

These are people who fail to grow up and instead get 'stuck' in a childish state of development. They can be undersized mentally, emotionally and physically. They can be tall and emotionally immature. There can be delayed development of physical organs, and overgrowth of tonsils is common, with accompanying mouth breathing and frequent colds.

As children they can be very shy, hiding behind their mothers' skirts, and generally slow to talk, walk and grow. They are often simple, small, or narrowminded and slow in understanding. Childish thoughts, repetitive simple talk, simple ideas, lots of irrelevant detail and care about little things are all common. The picture becomes more common in old age.

They cope with a simple life but complications send them into a dither of indecision. They fear strangers, new situations and being laughed at, which happens because of others' reactions to them, and they learn to cope by being silent in company.

Naive and simplistic are keynotes. They take advice and naively follow it. They can easily become dependent and are easily influenced. There is an extreme lack of confidence and a feeling of inferiority. They bite their nails.

In spite of all this they can grow up and, with considerable effort and strong narrow ability, achieve proficiency in such professions as science or medicine; but still the essential nature remains.

Trauma as disease

Backwardness. Tonsils swollen chronically, glands also hard. Second childhood in old age. Smallness of parts, e.g. testicles. Premature baldness. Headaches at school time.

BELLADONNA

Keyword **Red**
Source **Deadly nightshade**

Belladonna is frequently a remedy for acute fever illnesses with strong signs and great intensity, like red-hot fevers, hammering headaches, dilated, staring pupils, a fiery red face, a dry hot mouth, tongue and throat and dreams of fire. Pains are throbbing, shooting, cutting, sharp and right-sided. A keynote is a very hot head and body with cold hands and feet.

It is also a common chronic remedy for great intensity of symptoms.

Stresses

My guess is that they were given aspirin to suppress fever in childhood. Also violent abuse. Fevers are a natural process like breathing and aspirin is exactly the wrong treatment.

Attitude

Violence without sexual connections. Frequent behavioural problems. Heat to the head and cold to the feet, physically and emotionally. They are 'hot-blooded' emotionally and have 'cold feet' about life, being easily embarrassed and laughing loudly and smiling too much; the sort of people who have paroxysms of loud laughing at every opportunity. They can smile a lot, especially at the ends of sentences.

They tend to bubble away on the surface, while somatizing their feelings into their head. This can cause sudden complaints, sudden irritability, sudden anger, perhaps with increased strength, sudden biting, kicking, spitting and weeping, rapid flushing and vehement expression. They can hit and kick, awake or asleep. They kick out in bed. The face flushes red hot with anger, rage, coughing and other symptoms and there is quick blushing from embarrassment.

They suffer from right-sided pounding headaches, made better by lying down in the quiet. As adults they have right-sided migraines, right-sided severe throbbing headaches, right-sided facial paralysis and period pains and want to lie down in the quiet in all these situations. They can have great pain, possibly dragging, during the period, which is worse for any motion, worse for walking, worse for pressure, and they want to lie down.

As children, they can particularly crave lemon, being able to drink neat juice. Generally as children they fear dogs.

Trauma as disease

Behavioural problems. Right-sided migraines and headaches. Very high fevers. Right-sided facial paralysis. Painful periods. Violent behaviour.

CALCAREA CARBONICUM

Keyword **Fat and slow**
Source **Chalk**

Stresses

Mostly from prolonged overexertion or overwork, mentally or physically. Overcome by seeing suffering and injustice, especially upset by horrible things, stories, events in the news, greatly upset by terrible tragedies happening to others, by plane crashes and boats sinking, as well as by rudeness, worries, grief and anticipation.

Fears, of which they have many, can also overwhelm them: fear of going mad, of insects, spiders, dogs, ghosts, poverty, dark, heights, cancer, ill health, death, accidents, evil, mice or rats. In children the fear is especially of horrible stories, ghosts and the dark which can bring on nightmares.

Attitude

Calcarea are easily spotted. They are almost always fat, square-shaped, with squarely crosshatched foreheads. Being overweight is always a problem for them; being slim is not an option. 'Fair, fat and flabby' is a phrase that has been unkindly attributed to them.

They like to make others happy. They are worse from any exertion and can perspire or become out of breath just from going upstairs. They are almost always cold and perspire easily (as children, they are hot until five years old or so, as are almost all children).

Children are slow to develop and are known as plodders. They have sweaty heads at night as babies (Silica is the same but the sweat smells sour) and are content to just sit and play where they are put. While they are slow they are often very bright and can be great thinkers. They are tortoises rather than hares.

They are seemingly happy, contented people who may struggle but get there in the end. They are reliable, solid and dependable. However, they can overwork; they will work until they are exhausted and become overwhelmed by it and give up. They are interested in such things as reincarnation.

There is a rare thin version of this remedy with a very wrinkled, crosshatched forehead.

They are obstinately slow to adjust and change throughout life. They are slow to adjust to going to sleep (forcing themselves to stay awake as infants), slow to adjust to new situations, slow to start, slow to finish, slow in study, slow to change their minds, and slow to adjust to excessive overwork which overburdens them.

Trauma as disease

Asthma, eczema, rheumatism. Tend to have colds as children. Obesity.

CANNABIS INDICA

Keyword **Giggles**
Source **Plant**

Stresses

There are two main types – people who act as if their spirit is not fully engaged with their body, and people who take too much of the cannabis drug. The out-of-the-body types need it even though they have never used the drug; the others need to stop taking it. It may be of use in helping addicts to stop should they wish to.

Attitude

The 'natural' types are not 'earthed', but rather halfway to heaven. They are often very psychically or clairvoyantly mobile with a great ability to pick up on things from other realms, such as beautiful music from planes of existence that are not known on this one. They can have visions of future events.

Things are described by the frequent use of the keyword 'beautiful' and its ugly sister 'horrible' and many similar superlatives. They frequently use superlatives about other people, parents or friends, idealizing them out of all reality. They can feel themselves to be the opposite: horrible, worthless, totally lacking in confidence and very sensitive to criticism.

They tend to laugh and giggle at the least thing and can seem extraordinarily happy people, flamboyant, lively, exciting. They complain especially that they feel they are in the wrong place; heaven is where they want to be. To them their real home is up there. In reality they have failed to get into their physical body and Cannabis will help them do that.

They can see only the very good or the very bad and cannot face the 'bad' state of this world; so they idealize parts of it. They can shift between heaven and hell, from bliss to depression, or be stuck in either. They can become suicidal and may try to take an overdose. Classical music will lift their spirits in depression, taking them off towards heaven again.

They may indulge in spiritual practices, which for them are psychopathological, as their purpose is to come into the present and learn to live in their bodies.

These people have a sense of unreality, their time sense is awry and they have delusions about the size of things. Their mind is hazy and they are very forgetful. Theories abound in their minds and they theorize about everything. They often love to dance and have a strong hunger.

The drug-taker types can seem as if they have to argue themselves out of every intellectual, theoretical box they have got themselves into. They apply complex logic to seemingly obvious situations, apparently unable to get there by the direct route.

Trauma as disease

Anaemia and period problems seem to be common.

CARCINOSIN

Keyword   **Ordered chaos**
Source   **Cancer tissue**

Stresses

There is a disease wounding pattern from a history of cancer which leaves an imprint on subsequent generations. It does not mean that the person with this imprint will get cancer, although some will and it is more likely if the imprint is clear.

Reproaches, reprimands, anticipation, grief, horrible things, sad stories.

Attitude

They are generous, dancing, sympathetic, lively people. Many diverse specific factors mark out this type: family history of cancer, leukaemia, Hodgkin's disease, TB, diabetes, lupus, rheumatoid arthritis. As children, they either had no childhood diseases, or had multiple or bad doses. Blue tinge to the whites of the eyes.

There may have been a serious illness early in life, like pneumonia. There are congenital abnormalities, retardation, and causeless long drawn out inability to sleep and causeless sleeplessness in children and babies.

Fastidiousness is strong, in the way of perfectly matched outfits, co-ordinated clothes, socks of exactly equal length. They seek perfection.

A history of domination by forceful parents or partners. Excessive self-control and a very strong sense of responsibility, connected to guilt. Sympathetic, affectionate. Love of storms. Very sensitive to criticism, offended easily and yielding by nature.

Great fear of cancer. Many moles and the face may be a distinctive coffee colour. In babies severe red nappy rash, like Medorrhinum.

They can be artistic, love to dance, love music and even in the womb they move to music, like Sepia. Both these remedies share the image of 'children dancing outside in a thunderstorm'. They like to travel, like Tuberculinum.

They can often have a series of exact keynotes of several common homoeopathic remedies yet the full picture of none of them. A superficial understanding may lead you to the wrong conclusion so beware! It is as if cancer deranges the normal patterns of healthy expression of trauma and mimics several others.

Keynotes

Better by the seaside, although sometimes worse. Better in the evenings. Sleep with their knees up to their chests. Better according to the phase of the moon. Ailments from anticipation.

Love of dancing, animals, travel, storms. Restlessness in children and a destructive tendency. Desire for butter. Blueness of the white part of the eyes and brownish, *cafe au lait* complexion, numerous moles. Sleeplessness even in children.

A family history of cancer, diabetes, TB in one parent or two grandparents would be potentially indicative.

History of prolonged fear.

Trauma as disease

Any disease where the above fits.

CAUSTICUM

Keywords   **Crippled with anxiety**
Source   **Slaked lime mixed with solution of potassium sulphate**

Stresses

Death of a child, relative or friend. Long drawn out grief. Nerves anticipating an event, overexcitement. Fear, fright and horrible stories. Worry about others – friends and especially their children. Worry about injustice, exploitation. Actual injustice.

Attitude

Long drawn out grieving processes that are devastating in effect. Intense concern for the welfare of others. Overprotective. Overbearing towards their children. Excessive control of their children, will not let them near anything vaguely dangerous. Overcautious.

Dependent but bossy and quarrelsome at home. Sympathetic out of anxiety. Fear and dread that something will happen. Compulsive rechecking.

Great concern for exploited people, leading them to become trade union leaders, revolutionaries, anarchists, moralists or activists.

Externalized anxiety. Paralysing anxiety leading to local or total paralysis or crippling. A deeper picture is one of hopelessness, worthlessness, weeping without cause, despair, wanting to die, lack of courage, great guilt, as suicidal tendencies if they have committed some crime.

They are sensitive to both heat and cold and prefer it in between.

They feel stuck in a situation of hopeless injustice, and may go into active rebellion where this is possible.

The child is likewise very sympathetic and aware of suffering and the teenager can become idealistic and rebellious.

Trauma as disease

Localized paralysis, according to the focus and depth of their projected anxiety. Loss of voice. Often bladder weakness, with urination from laughter, coughing or exertion.

Bell's palsy, numbness of the face. Ménière's disease. Multiple sclerosis. Dupuytren's contracture, shortening of the tendons.

Crippling anxiety creating paralysing deformative arthritis. Cannot walk on heels as they are too painful. Writer's cramp. Carpal tunnel syndrome. Warts on the fingertips.

CHAMOMILLA

Keyword **Fitful Anger**
Source **Chamomile plant**

Stresses

Anger is what really upsets them and they themselves can be angry. Teething and toothache where the pain is keenly felt. Being severely told off. Disappointment.

Attitude

Infants who are so much in pain that they drive their parents to despair, who are impossible to please, very irritable, whiny and crying. They want something, demand it and immediately throw it away. They demand to be carried and will not be put down. They do not know what they want. Red cheeks, especially one red cheek, and fever.

Trauma as disease

Earache, cough, colic, from anger. Toothache or most commonly teething. Green stool.

Any illness from anger where they get local heat. Very uncivil as patients.

CHINA

Keyword   **Fragile**
Source   **Tree bark, quinine**

Stresses

Leaking. Long periods of heavy loss of body fluids, such as heavy perspiration or heavy periods. Loss of lots of blood. Prolonged diarrhoea. Childbirth with excessive loss of fluids. A severe debilitating illness.

Easily hurt by anything, very oversensitive to touch, motion, cold air, odours or the environment.

Children of parents who had malaria and were treated with quinine.

Attitude

Introverted, idealistic, very excitable and extremely touchy or irritable, especially in teenagers. Fear of dogs.

They have great fantasies especially at night and build castles in the air. Weakened and enveloped in self-protective apathy. They feel unfortunate and complain that they are hindered in their work by some person or organizational difficulty. They can feel rejected, unloved and persecuted and can blame others for their own misfortune.

Leaking emotionally and physically. Artistic. Great weakness after debilitation from above causation. Periodic complaints.

Trauma as disease

Anaemia. Wind, bloating and gas. Drenching night sweats. Profuse, never-ending periods. Debility.

COLOCYNTHUS

Keyword   **Colic**
Source   **Bitter apple**

Stresses

Greatly upset by the distress of others. Anger with indignation or silent grief. Bad news. Disappointment. Mortification. Taking offence.

Attitude

Typically colic of an infant when the parents are angry, which seems to happen often, and especially when there has been an episiotomy. Here the mother also needs Staphisagria.

A baby who gets colic every time a parent is upset.

Trauma as disease

Stomach ache from bitter apples. Colic or neuralgia with great pain from suppressed anger or vexation. Sudden, atrocious cramping, griping, tearing, cutting, pinching, clamping, gnawing, boring pains. Relief from doubling up, wriggling or hard pressure.

Cough and any acute symptoms from anger. Colic of

gallbladder (gallstones), in the ureter (kidney stones) and the uterus (dysmenorrhoea). Neuralgia and sciatica.

HYOSCYAMUS

Keywords   **Shocking and revealing**
Source   **Henbane plant**

Stresses

Jealousy. Sexual abuse. Anticipatory nerves. Disappointment in love and unhappy love. Admonition.

Attitude

Shamelessness and shocking are the threads that run right through this remedy, focused on sexuality. They may express this in sexually explicit ways, in obscenity and in pornography. For example, they can be embarrassingly frank when talking about personal things.

They use nakedness as a form of shocking, like the child who goes to the toilet and leaves the door open so they can be seen, or streakers, flashers, people who frequent nudist beaches or wear revealing clothes. They like being sexually shocking and offensive, in dress, in pictures, in drawings, in actions, to disturb and gain attention.

They use sexual jokes and pranks in inappropriate situations and sexual innuendo abounds in their conversations.

A keynote is that their hand tends to gravitate to the genital area, inside their clothing in children although not so often in adults. Children will masturbate in front of visitors in order to shock and upset their parents.

These people have a high sex drive and easy arousal and are extremely jealous. They can kill from jealousy as adults and as children.

Together with jealousy comes aggressive behaviour and there are some children who strike, beat, bite, break and take off their clothes. The aggression is milder than in other behavioural remedy types but combined with the sexual nature it makes for a unforgettable character. They can be banned from the nursery because of their antisocial behaviour.

Maliciousness with deviousness is another related aspect. Their jokes can become malicious and nasty although initially they might just be silly pranksters with inappropriate behaviour, lewd jokes in the wrong setting, etc.

Also in children and paranoid types, there can be low muttering, whispering and silence, or there can be loquacity with rapid changes of subject and outrageous speech.

There is egotism expressed as a strong need to be the centre of attention. There can be suspicion degenerating into deep mental states of paranoia with many delusions. They can pick at their clothes or play with their fingers, faces or lips.

So when aspects of sexual shock, nakedness, masturbation, jealousy, muttering, bizarre tics, egotism, suspicion, sexual innuendo, pranks and deliberate antisocial behaviour all occur together, this is the answer!

Trauma as disease

Behavioural problems in children. Exposing themselves. Manic depression. Paranoia. Schizophrenia.

IGNATIA

Keyword **Sighing**
Source **St Ignatia's bean**

Stresses

Any recent grief. This is the main recent grief remedy, required in so many cases as to be a household necessity. Some people, including children, can almost die from grief and this remedy can often be the one to put things right. Disappointment is a key causation, especially romantic disappointment, and very often the person wants to be alone to cry. There is also anger, contradiction, reproaches, shame, mortification, embarrassment and fright.

The death of a child or parent is a very important trauma, as is being in the womb while the parents are in grief.

Attitude

This can be a romantic, idealistic person, cultured, refined and sensitive. The emotional oversensitivity of the patient makes them almost a disappointment 'waiting to happen'. Initially they suffer by a brooding silence.

They do not need support. They are capable people who grasp things quickly.

They have to cry alone. They weep with sobbing and a lump in the throat. Sighing is very characteristic in adults, especially in any significant or meaningful conversation.

These people can put on a hard front, appearing cold but suffering inside. The front can be rude, suspicious or challenging. Especially as teenagers they can be critical and insulting. They often do not eat fruit and fear birds.

Trauma as disease

Any complaint that comes on after grief, even terminal illnesses, if the posture fits or no other remedy does.

Compare with Causticum and Nat mur.

KALI CARBONICUM

Keyword **Backbone**
Source **Salt of tartar**

Stresses

Rigid control of feelings. Overwork.

Attitude

It is very difficult for these people to express feelings and they keep a strong check on their emotions. They have a strong sense of duty and stick to a rigid inner code of right and wrong, of ethics and rules.

They are very stoical. They do not notice the stress they are under until the situation is very severe indeed. They are upset by things outside their control, especially fear of diseases. There is stiffness on all levels. They are strongly controlling like policemen, prosecuting lawyers, accountants, people who go 'by the book'.

They suffer in silence and can appear devoid of emotions yet are sensitive inside. As husbands they can be frustrating to live with as they will not show emotion.

There is also the image of the Alexander Technique teacher – people who have weak backs and need to sit up properly, upright or osteopaths. They are correct, orthodox, conventional people with a strong sense of morality; dogmatic and prone to take the moral high ground, to want to do things right.

They hold everything inside until they crack physically, so illnesses come suddenly and can be severe. They tend to quarrel with their spouse or family but are too dependent to leave them. They complain to such an extent that you want to strangle them.

Other signs are bags under the eyes or baggy lids, sleeplessness and asthma typically between 2 and 5 a.m., or around this time, sensitivity to cold draughts, weakness of heart, back, limbs and mind, sweaty backache and weakness with characteristic stitching pains.

They can be dull drab people who are overanxious about their symptoms. Anxiety and fear are felt in the stomach, as are sudden noises. A mother may be impatient with her children.

They can also appear as weak-willed, flabby, sweaty and puffing with asthma. This can arise from bottled-up anger, which brings on the attack of asthma. The same strong control is there but it breaks down as they become ill and they begin to quarrel, whereas when well they withhold their criticism and reserve it for themselves.

Trauma as disease

Back and joint pains, arthritis, catarrh, asthma, peptic ulcers and cancer.

LACHESIS

Keywords   **Intensely talkative**
Source   **Venom of snake**

Stresses

Grief or disappointed love. Restriction of any type. Jealousy.
No sexual outlet.

Attitude

This person has a wonderful set of 'call signs'. First, they are
tremendously talkative and the words come out in a non-stop
stream; it can be difficult to get a word in edgeways. They
seem to speak but not to listen. They are full of their own
ideas which they need to express so strongly that they are
described as compelling. A conversation with them seems like
a one-way process. Often you start a conversation and then
desperately try to find a way to end it politely; you change the
subject only to be subjected to another barrage of words.
Changing from subject to subject is common. They can be
sharp, witty, sarcastic and cutting in speech.

One positive aspect to their facility with speech is that they
can learn foreign languages quickly and they love to sing.

Everything about them is intense. If they are anxious they
are very anxious, about their health for example – enough to
make you think they are Arsenicum. A strong confirmation
can be achieved by getting them to stick their tongue out. It
will tremble like a snake's. There are other remedies that do
this but this is the main one. Another confirmation is their
fear of snakes.

Another useful feature is that they have left-sided complaints and the snake Lachesis has all its organs in the left side
of its body. In addition to this, the complaints go from left to
right, especially sore throats.

Lachesis women will get better immediately their periods
start – not just on the same day, like many women, but immediately. They are normally cold, although they can be hot,

but more importantly they suffer from rising heat and rising sensations, especially hot flushes to the head in numerous situations including menopause and just before puberty.

Another great feature is their jealousy. They can be insanely jealous all their lives; even when in a happy marriage they can still remain jealous without cause. This can develop into great suspiciousness and later paranoia. As young children they can be very jealous of their siblings, perhaps initially for good reason, but it does not wear off. Jealousy towards a new-born sibling may turn into asthma. Jealousy is anger mixed with sexuality and anger stored in the lungs often manifests as asthma. The child may say he 'hates' his new sibling; 'hate' is the call sign of Nat mur, but it is not as forcibly expressed as it is here. The child will actually say he hates the younger brother or sister and can be obviously revengeful.

As older people they can have cramps in the heart, high blood pressure, angina and palpitations and be unable to sleep on the left side as it aggravates the heart pains and palpitations.

They are often egotistical and can be arrogant.

There is an introverted type of Lachesis. They have a strong sense of inferiority and are very critical towards others. They seem to find and criticize the worst things in those around them; they can only see the bad things. This introverted type has a lot of envy, frustration and timidity.

They hate restriction of any sort, such as clothing around the neck; if they must wear a tie it is always loose. They dislike pressure and touch; they hate parental authority for the same reason and they often find the idea of marriage unendurable, again because of the idea of restriction. A keynote is pulling at clothing around the neck.

Keynotes

Fear of snakes – cannot even watch them on TV. Fear of heart disease. Like alcohol but later in life even a little upsets them or violently aggravates them.

Said to be hot but in my experience are cold people subject to hot flushes which they dislike intensely.

Worse after sleep. Better immediately the periods start.

Left-sided complaints and especially left-to-right symptoms. Worse in the spring, sometimes autumn. Worse lying on the left side.

Purple or bluish colour to skin, mottled purple. Red face as if about to burst, with a snakelike appearance. Aversion to touch.

Trauma as disease

Migraine headaches. Headache worse for heat and before periods. Flushes of heat to the face, especially at menopause. Otitis media, left side. Tonsillitis. Difficulty swallowing.

Gastrointestinal problems. Kidney stones. Nephritis. Ovarian cysts, left side. PMT.

Asthma. Wakes with suffocating feeling at night, especially on falling asleep. Hypertension. Cerebral accidents. Hemiplegia. Angina. Congestive heart failure. Myocardial infarction with constriction in chest, pain radiates to the left arm. Palpitations, worse lying on left side. Sleeps on right side, impossible on left.

LYCOPODIUM

Keywords **Blowing in the wind**
Source **Spores of club moss**

Lycopodium comes from the pale yellow spores of club moss, also known as stag's horn, which were used as a dusting powder for medicinal pills in the past as they are inert. However, potentization makes them into a powerful medicine. Aeons ago Lycopodium was a great treelike plant; it has shrunk down to a tiny moss as evolution progressed. The spores are not made wet by water but float on it. They are odourless and tasteless. Lycopodium is found in dry woods.

Homoeopathic Lycopodium, like all the remedies, mirrors the characteristics of the source. In this case they love power and appear big and dominating, like a stag's horns, a symbol of male supremacy, when they are feeling small and feeble inside, although they often do not realize it. Or they are just small and feeble and do not show the other side. They can be intellectually dry and dusty and have a lack of feeling, like the spores. They are unemotional. Lycopodium is an important liver remedy and yellow is the skin colour in liver disturbances.

Stresses

Stress, wounded pride, dented ego, humiliation, disappointments, betrayals, suppressed anger with silent grieving, domination by others, literary failure, things to do with a wounded, fragile ego.

Attitude

They are well known as dictators in their work or at home but at the other end of the scale can be very timid in all situations. They commonly display both traits in differing situations.

Their love of power makes them poor team players as they prefer to be at the top. Being essentially ambitious academics rather than practical types, they are found in professions rather than business, often at the top of a partnership or committee. They think they are equal players but to everyone else they act like the boss. They give the idea of a petty tyrant rather than a warlord.

They can be timid in all circumstances and present as extremely cautious people who feel pressurized by the least thing. They may like to teach yet feel very timid and lack confidence. You may not see any sign of assertiveness.

They can be tyrannical children and even before they speak they boss the parents around. 'He's the boss,' the parents may jokingly say about their six-month-old baby. When older, they can take the lead role and tell the others what they are doing wrong. They can correct what the parents say and seem to dominate them. Or they can be the introverted type, cautious and fearful of normal playground behaviour, and can become absorbed in safe, intellectual activities such as reading or computers. According to their type they can be either the bullied or the bully.

As adults they can have a classic low time around late afternoon and pick up later and get a 'second wind'. Wind, however, is what they frequently suffer from; distension of the abdomen is a definite keynote of this remedy. They are windy in the stomach and windy in speech, even dry and boring. Symbolized by the bagpipes, they drone on and on.

Cowardice is a word that often characterizes Lycopodium, especially a fear of people, based on a projection of their own inferiority.

Stress is another feature for this is really a how they experience their anticipatory anxieties and their fears of others. So they will classically complain of stress, which to homoeopaths is a 'dustbin' word covering a wide range of options and needs to be unfolded by simple questions like 'What exactly do you mean by stress?'

Commitment is a major issue for Lycopodium, because they find that their passion is shortlived; so they can thrive on affairs but not easily in marriage. The man may decide not to marry; or once the children have arrived and he is no longer top of the list in his wife's affections, he may run off with his secretary, who restores him to top place and massages his ego projections. One problem that can plague him is his anticipatory anxieties and his cowardice underneath, leading to failing erections.

Lycopodium as a remedy is subtle and the person may not notice it acting. Usually they become more confident but you have to ask their spouse about this; the patient probably will not realize it has done anything. It is common in males and in masculine women with seemingly overdeveloped academic intellect and lacking femininity.

Keynotes

Bossy to those they have power over, timid to those who have power over them.

Right-sided symptoms indicating that the male side of the personality is in distress, or right going to left, especially in acute illnesses.

Their low period is approximately 4 to 8 p.m. Often they say that their low time is around 4 p.m. and you have to ask

'And do you pick up again?' to confirm that they improve around 8 p.m. They can get a second wind then, becoming mentally active in the late evening.

They can be bad on waking.

They can either feel full as soon as they have eaten a little, or eating can stimulate a large appetite (reflecting again the small or large ego). Typical of the type is the intellectual student who comes home with a large bag of washing to be done for him or her, and who requests a snack and then consumes the contents of the fridge. They have a desire for sweets.

Rarely, one foot is hot, the other cold.

Trauma as disease

Any complaints where the above fits. Wind and gas, farting especially. Irritable bowel syndrome, meaning stress drives them to need to pass stool.

Tension. Stress-related complaints. Impotence from anticipation.

MEDORRHINUM

Keyword **Wild**
Source   **Gonorrhoea**

Stresses

Gonorrhoea in parent or grandparent, including what is called NSU. Excessive activity, too much indulgence in drugs, sex and excessive living.

Great nervousness before an appointment or once the time is fixed for something.

Jealousy.

Gonorrhoea

This is the most common sexually transmitted disease and results in urinary discharges, inflammation of the urinary organs, narrowing of the urinary tubes, inflammation of joints – knees, ankles, wrists, elbows – which are intractable, inflammation of the heart valves, severe conjunctivitis, swollen Bartholin's (vaginal) glands in women, inflamed fallopian tubes, recurring miscarriages, sterility, prolonged ill health, etc. This gives us a clear idea of its area of physical action.

There is a clear line of progression from suppressed discharges to rheumatoid arthritis to endocarditis and from suppressed infant nappy area eruptions to asthma.

Attitude

These are people who try everything – drugs, activities, affairs. They are oversexed, 'over the top' night people who feel at their best in the evening. There is an aggressive biting of the fingernails. They love the seaside or are better on holiday by the sea.

They sleep most comfortably on their front. They can be extremely jealous and hurried. They love animals even if they are allergic to them.

The essence of Medorrhinum is a somewhat excessive person who is larger than life, slightly coarse and crude and lacking in sensitivity. They are extrovert, do everything to excess if they can, are slightly wild and generally very lively.

They suffer from anticipatory anxiety over exams and important meetings, suffer greatly from hayfever and indulge dramatically in guilt. They tend to exaggerate everything and are larger than life.

There is a wildness and a hurriedness, a confused, scattered, unfocused mind. Their words may seem to be hidden behind a veil or a glass wall, and they may feel unreal, as if in a dream. They can have an abundance of ideas but no clear plan of what to do.

Procrastination is a common trait. They may have a poor memory.

Given a focus they can go to extremes; common excesses are pets, sex, work, extroversion or introversion, risk taking and drugs. This can lead to chaotic states.

Sex is the original cause of the infection (gonorrhoea) and sex is often the pointer. They focus on sex, and may be promiscuous: lots of sex in lots of positions with every type of partner. Sex can begin at the age of two, they can be living with a partner at fifteen and be worn out by sixty after several major operations.

They can oscillate between niceness and nastiness, between confidence and timidity, between cruelty and kindness, kicking the cat then stroking it, although they can have a real fear of cats.

These people have a fitful nature, spending energy in outbursts, so sporadic activities suit them best. Sustained energy is not for them.

As babies they can fail to thrive, wasting away, and very characteristically they can have a bright red nappy rash that is continuous over an area, like a scald. In bad cases this can appear elsewhere such as the face. They can be asthmatics. They can also lie on hands and knees, with their bottoms in the air, and sleeping like this at two years plus is a sign of this remedy.

These children are very sensitive to criticism, weeping when reprimanded, feeling that they must have committed some dreadful crime. They can be hard to manage at any age.

Keynotes

Extreme timidity. Extreme extroversion. Fear of the dark. Fear of someone behind them. Fear of insanity.

Compulsive hand-washing. Aggressive nail-biting.

Clairvoyance (prophesying disagreeable events) which they deny. Great sensitivity of the soles of the feet in rheumatism.

They are night people, and come alive then. They love being by the seaside. They sleep on the front or in the recovery position.

Intense cravings for oranges and orange juice, unripe fruit, salt, sweets and fat. Aversion to peas.

Hairy arms. Menses stain indelibly. Hasty aggressive speech, even when being friendly.

Wildness and need to experience everything. Partners in several towns. Jealousy leading to knife fights.

Dreams so real they believe them. Early masturbation.

Retarded children with masturbation and red rashes, even on the face. Egotism when older and wildly successful.

Hot feet they stick out of bed.

Trauma as disease

Bright red nappy rashes when a parent has had some sexual infection. Fishy smelling thrush or other discharges. A lot of catarrh which sticks in the throat and has to be hawked up. Thick catarrh in nose.

Asthma where they are best on their knees and chest in bed. Discharges from birth. Hayfever. Warts anywhere. Early onset of heart disease. Reiter's syndrome. Nail-biting with asthma.

MERCURY

Keyword   **Reactive**
Source   **The metal**

Stresses

Vulnerable to being obstructed by something like a legal suit or a business problem.

Suffer from betrayal, rejection, disappointment and sexual excess.

Attitude

Basically very sensitive to everything. If you welcome them in and make them feel very secure they will open up and blossom, whereas as soon as they notice the slightest negativity they close up and stay that way. So like the mercury thermometer, they take the emotional temperature of every situation and react exceedingly quickly. This is their call sign. When they close up they can exhibit trembling and stammering, which stop when they are relaxed. So they can seem to be extremely closed, cautious and suspicious by nature (such people may look out of the corners of their eyes).

When they bond they do so tightly, which can lead to sexual excesses. They are flirtatious, especially children, and precocious. Inside they feel hurried all the time, often believing they cannot cope and feeling overwhelmed.

They are very conservative people who need a stable life to counter their inner state of disunity. They are discontented, lack confidence, are sensitive to criticism and go on to hate the offending person, which can lead to violent impulses.

They crave bread and butter, dribble a lot as infants, and may stutter.

Mercury

Mercury is like electric jelly, so these people are sensitive, impulsive and trembling. It is the heaviest liquid and the only common liquid metal. It needs a very strong surface tension to hold it together on a flat surface, so it has tremendous internal conflict between inner pressure and outer surface tension. The person may have delusions of being surrounded by enemies and of being at war within and without. There are many feelings of paranoia and separation.

Mercury was called the chameleon mineral in the past as it reflects its surroundings like a mirror. So these are tricky people who reflect the outside situation, their surroundings, not who they are.

On a flat surface mercury splits into many parts if it is disturbed and is very unstable without a strong container. Mercury people are therefore very easily disturbed by outside influences. They are unstable and impulsive, cannot find a place to be, physically or psychologically, and are impossible to tie down.

The substance forms amalgamations with other metals, needing a stabilizer, so once they bond the person will stay in strong associations for life.

Trauma as disease

Recurring ear problems as infants; otitis media. Tooth and gum problems. Ulcerative colitis. Parkinson's disease.

NATRUM MUR

Keywords   **Responsible helper**
Source   **Salt**

Stresses

The main woundings to these vulnerable people are from disappointment, especially disappointed love and long-felt and remembered disappointments.

They suffer grievously from many of life's tragedies, as well as from any form of criticism, especially humiliation, and rejection, betrayal, anticipatory stress, bad news, fright, ridicule and scorn.

Attitude

Nat murs exist in all walks of life as natural responsible people or professional helpers and they are great listeners but poor sharers of their own feelings. You can have a Nat mur friend for years and still not know them. They are very private people. Closed is a word that describes them well and secretive is another. They often seem strong to others as they do not divulge their own weakness.

They can often, but by no means always, function well in society, at home, school and works with a very sociable front, and can communicate well intellectually as effective pro-fessionals, but they are exceedingly vulnerable inside emo-tionally and are afraid to let their feelings show in case they are hurt. This type of person is very common in western society. Being locked into this posture means that they fail to learn from experience the value of sharing. They can stay closed all their lives.

The main hurts these vulnerable people experience are from disappointment, especially in love. In fact as they can be so easily hurt, every insult experienced by Nat mur can be held against the offender a long time, often for ever. Classic-ally they say things like, 'You get over it but never forget it' when talking of some deep grief or loss, as if this is the only possibility. They really believe this to be true, as it is their experience. Taking Nat mur will change this experience.

'Hate' is a key word for them, based on long-remembered insults, although it usually means just 'dislike'.

Nat murs rarely cry and if they do, they do it in private, seeing crying in front of others as a humiliation. Often their eyes show long-suffering sadness and a need to cry. When they do cry, they hate sympathy and consolation and want to be left alone.

Blocked tears cause symptoms that act as substitutes, like hayfever which can be understood as alternative tears.

Nat mur mothers generally discourage tears in their children by distraction or ridicule or simple things like 'There, there, don't cry' messages, conditioning the child to believe tears are not an acceptable form of expression.

As responsible mothers and fathers Nat murs tend to show care and material support without sufficient cuddles and expressed loving. In fact Nat mur fathers can show no affection at all yet love their child.

They tend to adopt a position of responsibility early in childhood. They are often the oldest child or the girl who helps the mother with her younger siblings. They learn early on that this is a way of gaining approval, a poor substitute for love but the best on offer.

As teenagers, perhaps after an early disappointment which hurts them tremendously, they are reluctant to have partners out of a fear of further rejection, and can isolate themselves in safe activities such as reading, music, etc. They may also isolate themselves by sitting apart in groups and classes and tend to want to be alone a lot. They can become serious, unable to take or make jokes, introverted and isolated, seeking not to hurt or be hurt. They can appear cold and distant. At school they are good pupils, doing well, seeking to please perhaps, and are responsible about homework. They are easy to discipline as even slight disapproval is enough for them but they can need very sensitive handling to achieve any constructive criticism. Introversion describes them well at this stage – the watcher on the sidelines.

Later they can develop a posture of outward sociability, apparently at ease in society, but they never let anyone too close. Fathers of this type commonly do not express their feelings for their children and the children do not receive overt support, although they may learn that they are loved in other ways.

In adult life they are the classic responsible professional helper, the wounded healer, teacher, social worker, nurse, counsellor, writer, broadcaster, editor, secretary, etc. They seek to do their job to perfection to avoid criticism and hurt, so as employees they are very high-quality workers, but they are not good in positions of sharing and where negotiation is required.

Men can find it impossible to urinate in a stand-up urinal. Women and men both hate to be seen crying except perhaps at a film. Drinking relaxes them and they can then be un-inhibited as the control lessens and they let their hair down.

Nat mur men often run marathons (running away from their feelings, which they find it hard to contact?). They eventually collapse, perhaps with postviral weakness, and will not agree they are at all better until they can run a marathon again. In fact Nat murs are the worst patients, as even when they are clearly getting better by an objective criteria, they are still likely to say nothing has changed. They even keep getting better a secret.

Both sexes can fall in love with unavailable married people, which allows them to stay safe from reality. They will often have a lover living abroad or a long way away, at university, for example. This way they may get sex without closeness, which to them is threatening.

Keynotes

Above all else, they prefer salty things to eat. They hate meat fat, and will never eat it. They can like chocolate.

Headaches and migraines are their favourite complaints, as well as hayfever (alternative tears). They are worse from being in the sun, headaches especially.

They are closed, secretive and vulnerable, do not cry, except rarely and alone, and do not want any sympathy when they are upset. 'Hate' is a favourite word.

They remember insults for a long time, like the proverbial elephant. They take responsibility for others and are good listeners. They are quiet and withdrawn and watch others. They require harmony. They sit apart in groups and do not easily join in.

They fall in love with unavailable people and can be deeply attached without showing it. They grieve strongly without showing it, with many symptoms after grief.

They dislike noise, light, smoke.

Allergies and eczema. Divergent squint. Backache better lying on a hard surface. Claustrophobia. Fearful of burglars.

Trauma as disease

Headaches are their chief symptom, owing to incarcerated anger which explodes in their brain. The sun makes them worse, hating illumination (sympathy and kindness) as they are closed about their feelings.

This remedy cures more headaches than aspirin. I do not think it is an exaggeration to say that it is the world's greatest headache cure!

They can suffer from ME/postviral syndrome, MS and glandular fever especially when there is TB in the family.

Hayfever (alternative tears). Sleeplessness, from grudges left over from the day. Dryness of eyes, lips, mouth and vagina, dry skin, along with cold sores and cracked lips if they do not use a lip salve. (They must avoid camphorated lip salves for homoeopathy to work.) Herpes anywhere.

But like all the profiles, whatever the disease, if the profile fits you, it can cure anything, so try it.

NITRIC ACID

Keyword **Grudges**
Source **The chemical**

Stresses

Great sensitivity to emotional and physical pain, to jarring and touch, to little things like sad stories, to rushing about and excitement and to loss of sleep.

Discord between parents and children, between spouses or boss and an employee, or with neighbours.

Attitude

These people hold grudges even against their own will; they cannot forgive and forget. They are unmoved by apology, aggressively angry against perceived injustice, bearing the grudge until the day they die. They are pessimistic and critical, yet they can be very sensitive, refined, sympathetic, artistic, caring, concerned people. Conversely they can be selfish, self-absorbed, egotistical, hard to like, pests, cynical, quarrel-some, angry, distrustful, bitter and resentful.

They have great concern for their health, a despair of recovery, a fear of death, even suicidal thoughts. They will not be reassured, and are very concerned that the remedy will be counteracted by minor things.

They fear but long for death.

Trauma as disease

Acne (this is the No. 1 remedy). Splinterlike pains in inflamed parts including ulcer pains, pus pains and throat pains. Ulceration and ulcerative gnawing. Warts. Cracks in the skin.

NUX VOMICA

Keyword   **Businessman**
Source   **Plant (nut)**

Stresses

Anger is paramount in Nux vomica. Anger with indignation or silent grieving can be major exciting causes. Humiliation is particularly strong. Traumas from bad news, disappoint-ment, grief and taking offence occur too.

Deception, as may occur in a business deal or a job promotion done other than by the book, or professional jealousy, could be overwhelming. Deep deception, such as not being told you are adopted until much too late, can be almost mortally wounding and certainly life-changing.

Jealousy is also a strong causative factor, between children especially.

Since Nux vomica is a main remedy for business people, it is also a main remedy for people with problems relating to their business.

Attitude

Spasm is caused by the strychnine in the nut and characterizes much of their behaviour too. There is an intensity to their actions: spasms of anger and rage they cannot control, for example.

Nux vomica is the classic impatient, hardworking, driven business type. They can be small shopkeepers who work long hours, captains of industry, police, or military officers, any hardworking ambitious professionals who act as well as think as a basic posture in life. They are very sensitive to their surroundings, being easily irritated by anything – noise, light, touch, odour or slight pain. Any delay sparks their temper. On the phone or face to face they are direct, demanding and forthright. They are irritated by obstruction of their purpose, ambitious and often highly sexed. They are chilly people.

The type is more male than female, but certainly can fit both. They tend to be slim and muscular.

Keynotes

Strongly ambitious, ruled by goals and seeking to achieve. Fear of marriage and of intimacy.

Irritable and impatient, cannot abide queuing, curse other drivers. Critical and fastidious. Aggressive and quarrelsome as a habit. Strong sexual energy.

Chilly people, addicted to coffee, alcohol, stimulants. Wake at 4 a.m.

Sensitive to noise, odours, light, touch, pressure of clothes, especially around the waist.

Trauma as disease

Ulcers, any gastric upsets, constipation, cramps, irritable bowels, hayfever, repeated bouts of sneezing, hernias, cystitis, headaches, hangovers, etc.
Constipation, with a feeling that they have not finished after a stool.
Feeling of a stone in the stomach.

PHOSPHORIC ACID

Keyword **Apathetic**
Source **The chemical**

Stresses

Excess of narcotics, drug abuse, debilitating illnesses. A very repressed person who suffers silently from anger with silent grieving, especially over the death of a child, and disappointment, especially in love.
Fright. Homesickness. Humiliation. Too much excitement.

Attitude

These people are apathetic, burnt out, slow to answer, worn out, tired, with no feelings at all. Nevertheless, they can work long hours as passive workhorses. They are worse than Sepia. They crave refreshing fruit and drinks.

Trauma as disease

Hair falling out and going grey early. Apathy.

PHOSPHORUS

Keyword   **Friendly**
Source   **The chemical**

Stresses

Too impressionable. Lots of friends, and tending to an excessive concern for others. They exhaust themselves by a process of diffusion of energy.

Attitude

Phosphorus is flamboyant, often with red, white or black hair. They are outgoing, open people who are naturally kind and considerate to others, although they may appear indifferent because of 'sympathy exhaustion'. They are lively, creative, artistic and musical; this is the first remedy to think of for all artists. They tend to have a sort of phosphorescent skin that radiates lightness. They are normally thin, attractive, affectionate, with bright eyes, long eyelashes and graceful movements, and they love life and living. They have many friends, often half a dozen good ones, and confide in them easily about everything. If a Phosphorus moves location they quickly form new friendship groups because of their ability to share easily and confide. The ability to make friends easily is a confirmation of Phosphorus.

As children they are very easy to spot. Thin, with an occasional tubby version, they give and receive affection unlike Pulsatilla which only takes it. They give kisses naturally and like stroking; they seem magnetized by it. They are usually good at drawing and also perhaps music and are generally of the artistic, refined type. They are lively, impressionable and attractive, with the common phosphorescent skin and warm nature.

Children are often scared of the dark, scared of ghostly stories and even disturbed by typical children's stories like 'Little Red Riding Hood'. Parents quickly learn about their sensitivities and their inability to sleep after frightening stories, television, etc. They will need to sleep with the hall light on and the door ajar, and although this is common in many children, here the fear of the dark is strong and persists beyond the normal age. It is not at all uncommon to find an adult Phosphorus still afraid of the dark, although this often turns into a fascination with the dark, ghostly stories, etc. as they grow up.

They are often very thirsty, craving cold drinks, and also ice cream, chocolate, burgers, fish, fizzy drinks and salty things. In craving salt and chocolate they are like Nat mur, yet they are the polar opposite in personality.

As teenagers we can find two common versions, one definitely reserved and shy and another still radiating and glowing. The latter is eager, enthusiastic, open, gullible, outgoing, artistic and aiming for art college, nursing or music, according to their kind, sympathetic nature and their particular artistic expression. The food cravings are the same but they prefer burgers and especially chocolate. They can easily burn out at this stage from dancing, late nights, etc. As they are often intelligent, they can do their homework easily and burn the candle at both ends.

Later on they may become more anxious and while still possibly fearful of the dark, have another fear which is spoken of as if 'something may happen' or words to that effect. It is not uncommon for their thyroid to misfunction, especially after giving birth. It burns out and they need Phosphorus to restore it. They can be anxious about their health but they respond to reassurance even over the telephone and their worst fears often then abate.

As the children leave home, Phosphorus parents can become overanxious about them, worrying unnecessarily, and also worrying excessively about their own health.

Numbness in the fingers and toes can occur and at any stage in life easy bleeding of bright red blood is possible, as are burning pains anywhere, like the flame from phosphorus. In particular, the chest is their weak point and coughs, burning pains, acute chest complaints, colds that go to the chest, sputum streaked with fresh blood, tight chests and oppressed breathing will respond to Phosphorus, given this personality.

Keynotes

Open, extrovert or reserved. Creatively artistic in some form. Kind and sympathetic.

Often tall, thin and delicately boned. Occasionally very tall and graceful with it. Red, white or jet black hair that is natural and shines.

Cravings for chocolate, salt, cold drinks, fizzy drinks, ice cream, burgers, fish, chicken. Dislike tomatoes (not the same as tomato ketchup, which they may like).

Fear of the dark. Scared and cannot sleep after ghostly stories, television, etc. Like and need company. Form friendships easily. Sparkle like phosphorus and glow.

Anxiety about their health when older. Anxiety about others when adult. Like a tea bag in a hot bath, they diffuse and become exhausted because of their kindness, anxiety and sympathy, so boundary-making is important for them.

Phosphorus

This is the substance that matches are made of. When you light a match it flares up, is very hot, radiates light, burns brightly and then goes out, turns to dark ashes. Phosphorus people are very similar. They light up easily on meeting people, radiate warmth, give out kindness and loving feelings and burn out as quickly if they have not mastered the art of slow burning, becoming more like a candle. They can fade, lose their energy and colour, and go pale and grey.

PLATINA

Keyword **Haughty**
Source **The metal**

Stresses

Wounds to the ego. Hurt by anger, especially associated with fright and worry, and by scorn or contempt. Disappointment, especially sexual, and deceived ambition.

Emotions, touch.

Attitude

They are haughty, self-loving, contemptuous, arrogant, proud, dominating and superior. They see others as small. These things are shown in jests like 'I treat them like little boys, these so-called grown up men'. Such throw-away lines frequently indicate the underlying state.

They exhibit extremes of sexuality, exploring all types of sex. They are easily sexually excited and often masturbate.

They go to extremes, with high drama, an air of mystery and seductiveness. Relationships are tumultuous, with great intensity and jealousy, but shortlived.

They have fleshy prominent lips. They are idealistic, bear grudges and feel deserted, separated, divided and isolated. They can be depressed, but are better in the open air.

Trauma as disease

Numbness of head and lips, Bell's palsy, numbness of sexual area, general numbness. Bandaged feeling. Local coldness. Ovarian cysts.

PULSATILLA

Keywords   **Attention-seeking**
Source   **Wind flower**

Stresses

Rejection or feeling that they are rejected, unloved and unwanted is their major trauma. Everything revolves around this. An enforced separation from the mother directly after birth is a likely cause, or a parent who is absent early on in their lives. They may feel that they are not, or never were, loved enough and this may be true. Betrayal is likewise a strong wounding.

They can also be hurt by fright, grief, bad news, humiliation and disappointment, and be upset by overexcitement.

Attitude

The images of the pussy cat and the barking dog both summarize Pulsatilla well. As the pussy cat they love stroking, appreciation, attention and almost purr, soaking it up as a child and perhaps all their life, seeking attention by sitting in their mother's lap, especially if another sibling wants it. They seek to be No. 1 in the lap, in attention, in cuddles.

Later they can manipulate for attention with their favourite comment, 'Do you love me?'. As the dog, they can be very narrowminded, fixed in their attitude, seeking attention, fanatical, dogmatic, with a one-track message. This dogmatic one-track approach is founded on the insecurity of abandonment which was the formative experience of their lives. Separation at birth, a disappearing parent, an absent father, the early death of a parent – one of these is frequently at the root.

Being single-minded and seeking company, women can easily become mothers at an early age. They can be the archetypal mother, wanting lots of babies to fill the abandonment void, and can have milk in their breast even when not breastfeeding, as the sight of another baby can bring it back. They are very cuddly and attentive to their children, but can easily become overprotective, overcompensating for their own traumas.

This is all tied in with gaining attention to satisfy their deep, seemingly insatiable need. They want pity. Yielding and submissiveness are very common yet combined with the manipulative behaviour they often help the person get their own way. The child clings to its parents, the wife to her husband.

Being essentially stuck in a childlike state they can naturally weep at the drop of a hat, and they can easily put it on. As they get older they may put up a hard front and hide the weeping, but underneath it is the same, with the same attention-seeking strategy. And they weep when angry too; the two are frequently confused in Pulsatilla. They can be very friendly people, concerned and wanting to be involved.

Jealousy is common in a mild way, mildness being another characteristic. A changeable nature is common; their moods change frequently and you have to assess which one is current every time you meet them.

They are hot people who are generally thirstless. They may say that they have to force themselves to drink. They blush easily and must have fresh air. They are plump, often fair, easily jealous and fear going mad.

They crave sweets, butter and cheese and hate fat, which disagrees with them, and pork. They get indigestion from ice cream and especially fatty things.

Children and adults both sleep on their backs with their hands above their heads, or on their fronts.

Pulsatillas become very dependent and so find it hard to leave relationships. They are tidy people, often from a sense of disgust, and this can lead to obsessive cleanliness.

Evenings and mornings are bad times for Pulsatilla.

Open air always helps. They are frequently seen sitting near windows and stuffy cafes are no-go areas.

Keynotes

Thirstless. Warm people needing lots of fresh air.

Seek attention, want company. Feel abandoned.

Dislike all fat. Like sweets. Jealous. Weepy and like consolation. Yellow discharges.

Dogmatic and manipulative.

Trauma as disease

In infants glue ear, thick yellow discharges, yellow matter coming out of the inner corners of the eyes.

Mild earache, whining and wanting to be carried. Stomach or headache at school time (feeling of rejection and manipulation in full unconscious swing). Weeping when mother leaves them at the nursery.

Diseases like mumps and measles affecting breasts and testicles. Light and short periods. Painful and stinging varicose veins especially in pregnancy. Inflamed chilblains. Later, wandering arthritis. Swelling of knees.

Sleeplessness from one thought repeating. Lots of heart pains, anxieties felt in the heart and a fullness usually in the evenings. Lots of moles. Blocked noses.

SEPIA

Keywords **Needs to dance**
Source **Ink of the cuttlefish**

Stresses

These people feel most of their troubles in the sexual area which is their most vulnerable spot. Suppressed anger, romantic disappointments, fright, bad news and being offended all affect them keenly, but what really strike home are abortions, having sex when they do not feel like it, which can be most of the time, and being worn out by their family, especially young children who will be very demanding because they find it very hard to be affectionate.

Attitude

As teenagers they are fairly undifferentiated, enjoying life and relationships, but later on they suffer a great deal from apathy and indifference to their husbands, children and relatives in general. Neutralized feelings, feelings of alienation and an inability to give affection are common attitudes. They are irritated by company and want to be alone, and are indifferent to sex. Their great release is through dance and physical exertion; these make them feel good and transforms their energy. It is their alternative expression of sexual energy.

As teenagers, they usually say that they enjoy sex provided they are getting on well with their partners; they are not the types for casual sex, which gives an early clue. They have seven-day periods and must exercise or dance daily.

If they are fair or red haired they can have clusters of freckles concentrated over the nose and cheeks, whereas

Phosphorus, another remedy with red hair that exhibits indifference, can have freckles on the nose only (like Sulphur).

They can have great insights into others, see weak spots and make cutting remarks. Later they can become 'guru-type' people full of detachment arising from their own unfeelingness.

This remedy is well known as the marriage reviver when one partner has drifted into this state out of exhaustion, and is fed up or run down, and especially when the mother wants to quit, leave her children and go off somewhere – the neutralized feelings can go that far.

They usually have to be occupied doing something – sewing, DIY, knitting – even while watching TV.

Sepia children love thunderstorms and dancing.

Sepia has an aversion to consolation and wants to cry alone. They may have herpes on the lips or cracked lips.

It is possible to confuse Sepia with Nat mur, but the difference is to be found in Sepia's love of dance and Nat mur's love of salt, and the general demeanour.

Trauma as disease

Frigidity, lack of sexual enjoyment, sterility and spontaneous abortions are all common from reduced energy in the sexual region. Men are similar.

Dryness of vagina. Thrush is very common, even in young girls. Heavy long periods. Any number of period problems. PMT.

Backache. Vitiligo. Hot flushes at the menopause.

SILICA

Keywords   **Yielding but persisting**
Source   **Flint**

Stresses

Stress, exams, performing in public, new situations especially, failure, being told off, ridicule, wounded pride, fright, excessive sexual activity, excessive mental activity.

Vaccinations (except smallpox – see Thuja).

Attitude

Yielding but resilient is one of the catchphrases of this remedy. Yielding, lacking the grit for doing the job, dreading failure, faint-hearted, retiring, shirking, wavering, uncommitted, spineless, avoiding confrontation passively, timid, shy and very cautious are other descriptions.

They hate to argue and confront yet, being very stubborn, will not give way, so they slide off in some way and avoid conflict without resolving the issue. A child will go to another room to avoid conflict with a parent and do what the conflict is about behind the parent's back.

A basic concept in this remedy is a failure to express and receive. Silicas cannot expel pus from abscesses, splinters (the remedy is good for doing just this) or stools; they find it hard to express themselves or to assert themselves, with slowness as a keynote. At the same time they fail to assimilate food, have poor nutrition and weak nails and hair, are slow to assimilate ideas and have to study long and hard. This slowness to assimilate exists at all levels, with resilience and stubbornness and persistence as intermediaries.

The Silica type becomes a bright, able, intelligent student and a high achiever at school. Studying can become a way of life, and they can avoid the real world and become eternal students. They can go from school to college to lecturer to professor. However, various symptoms result from all the studying they have to do to achieve, with mental exhaustion from excessive reading and writing and going blank beyond a certain point. There is a similar 'blankness' on other levels: a bald head, especially the vertex, white spots on nails and teeth, dullness, etc.

This type is a professional rather than a business person, as the former has a less aggressive occupation. They are not natural leaders as they lack the courage, but may get into leadership positions reluctantly. They like to be valued usually in an academic or professional way and carve out a career by being appreciated for their image, for example as the devoted professional, the studious learned scholar who writes books.

They are also successful people who swerve out of the fast lane, the chairman or TV producer who becomes a postman or organic gardener.

A Silica child speaks to you only with the mother as intermediary, too shy to talk directly.

Keynotes

Fear needles and the dentist because of injections. Therefore not keen on acupuncture either. Anticipatory anxiety.

Babies averse to mother's milk, with big heads, thin bodies (poor assimilation), reluctant sour stools and open fontanelles, and a sour-smelling perspiration of the head.

Early baldness in the intellectual type, vertex and elsewhere. White spots on most fingernails, nails break easily, ingrown toenails. Sweaty, smelly feet and fungus between toes. Receding chin.

Aversion to bright colours. Limp handshake. Strongly sensitive to the moon.

Trauma as disease

Headaches from the back of head extending to the forehead. Stubborn festering wounds. Abscesses of long standing. Enlarged glands. Easy scarring. Acne leaving scars. Mental exhaustion from excessive study, which they are prone to do.

Frequent recurring infections. Frequent ear infections in children. Hard glands.

This remedy is slow to act, as are the patients, so wait a few weeks or months before deciding it has worked.

STAPHISAGRIA

Keyword **Suppression**
Source **Plant**

Stresses

Suppression and non-expression of anger. Rape. They feel anger strongly but never express it. It is the classic doormat posture; however badly treated, they smile sweetly and continue to bear it. Or they live in a situation where anger cannot be expressed, typically with a violent husband.

This is the main victim remedy in assaults like rape where abuse and rage are paramount, not fear. In a rape with terrific violence Stramonium would be needed first and Staphisagria once the terror had been dealt with. The rage is held in the body structures around the offended place.

They also feel they have been assaulted after operations on sexual parts, like episiotomies or hysterectomies, when the body feels 'raped' but it has all been done under anaesthetic. Many women never have sex again after hysterectomies because they feel violated and hold a lot of suppressed anger in the sexual area. Making love brings up this pent-up rage but as these people repress their anger, they give up sex instead.

It is frequently needed for the mother after childbirth, when she feels assaulted. Attempted abortion can induce great rage in the foetus, who has no way to express it.

It is also needed for any complaint where anger is not dealt with or anger with indignation or silent grief suppressed, disappointments and disappointed love, indignation and mortification.

It is useful for people stuck in patterns of repeatedly being violated or people whose relationships are always with spouses that violate them.

On a more general level this remedy is often needed in countries and cultures where there has been endless suppression and colonization, or areas under the control of some outside power. It is also widely needed in countries where men have dominated women for centuries and they live apparently happily with repressed lives. It is needed in families where people are subject to excessive parental authority, not necessarily of the violent type but just where submission is the norm, and where the housing situation means several generations live on top of each other.

The key rubric here is causation from suppressed anger. All the above may therefore reflect a range of remedies, so it is important to make sure the picture below is also present.

Attitude

Staphisagria is a nice, sweet man or woman with a dominant spouse – a very common attitude in some countries – or with several women living together in one house, with Staphisagria as the doormat.

It also applies to any victim of an aggressor, where the aggression can just take the form of power rather than a threat.

They remain nice and smiling whatever the situation, based on trying the best they could as a child faced with a strict or violent parent and with no other defence, or based on religious ethics like turning the other cheek and smiling.

They tell you that they are terrible when they get angry. In fact they just throw things, slam doors and break things, but they feel that this is terrible. It is the child of strict parents who rushes outside and throws something in anger. Suppressed anger and throwing things when they finally crack sums it up.

Styes on eyelids is a clue as is early masturbation in children. Sexuality and masturbation are in proportion to the suppression of feeling.

Trauma as disease

Any complaint based on the above.

STRAMONIUM

Keywords   **Clinging from terror**
Source   **Plant**

Stresses

This is a major terror remedy, birth trauma terror being a very common causation, along with terrors from wars long past or recent. It can be needed several generations on from a war.

It is for terror that occurs whenever someone is trapped in a confined space, such as a birth canal, an incubator or a lift that is stuck. It is also for the terror of bombing.

Other causations are separations with prolonged *isolation* or short, critical isolations such as being left in an incubator unattended after birth, which can bring on terror, frightening anger, such as might be experienced from a violent father. Abortion being considered can be felt as violence by the foetus and can replay throughout the life.

It applies to children brought up in violent, alcoholic or fanatical religious families, where violence is common, and to people who went to schools where the cane was used indiscriminately.

It also applies to attacks by muggers and rapists or being held at gunpoint, where there is a threat of death, not just rape, and where the fear is paramount, to terror where death is a possibility or a near certainty and to attempted strangulation, where the victim becomes unconscious.

Attitude

These people have a great fear of violence or attack. They can also have violent fantasies and be aggressive, violent themselves, like muggers, soldiers who rape at gunpoint, people with violent impulses who have to restrain themselves from hitting their children and fathers who leave home for this reason as they cannot cope with the violence that their children bring out in them.

It also applies to people who find themselves in relationships with someone who is potentially violent or threatening or actually violent, yet whom they cannot leave because they also have a fear of abandonment.

Great fear of being alone at night is a keynote. They are so scared of the dark that even as adults they might have to sleep with the light on.

Stammering on the first word is another keynote.

They can be poets and songwriters in verse or singers who also write.

They can experience terrifying nightmares which wake them up with a wild look and they are almost inconsolable, especially babies and children after a delayed second stage of birth.

There is a fear of violence, deep water, shiny and reflecting surfaces, mirrors, even cassette tape, the dark, monsters, dogs, black dogs, dogs at night or being alone at night. They often wear black clothes and are fascinated by the dark but fear graveyards and crave light.

They also fear tunnels, especially if the train stops and the lights go out, and suffer from claustrophobia. As children they can kick, hit, bite, etc. like Belladonna but unlike Belladonna, they can be jealous, but the key thing is the night terrors, fearing to be alone at night, etc.

They can feel isolated and alone and compensate by clinging, for example always sitting in the same place to study in the library or being unable to drive as they cannot leave their base. They may cling to their spouse and say that they deeply love them, in a sense that makes clinging a better interpretation.

Religion can be a compensation for the deep feeling of isolation; God, after all, is everywhere to cling to.

Close to Aconite.

Trauma as disease

Convulsions. Stammering. Religious fanaticism.

Any complaint with these woundings and attitudes.

SULPHUR

Keywords   **Itchy inventors**
Source   **Mineral**

Stresses

Wounded pride or wounding of their inflated ego is their main stress; because of their self-centred nature nothing much else affects them, except embarrassment because it hurts their inflated ego. Bad news and horrible stories do get through. Derives from conditional loving by parents.

Suppressed anger creep out of their skin as itching (irritation) and eruptions (anger boiling over).

Attitude

The basic remedy has many facets to it but it has certain fixed characteristics that run through many different profiles.

There is almost always a history of skin eruptions that itch. There is an inquisitive, inventive nature. There is plenty of energy and often hyperactivity.

Egotism is present from the cradle to the grave. 'Me' is the centre of their universe; they are self-centred in the sense of always seeing others and things in relation to themselves.

They are lazy and untidy to the extreme; their room is a tip but they say they know where everything is!

They can have great hunger all the time and especially hunger for mid-morning snacks, at 11 a.m. to be precise, so they become fat. They may have a very sweet tooth and often dislike eggs.

They very commonly fear heights.

They are mostly very hot people, wear few clothes even in winter, and very often stick their feet out of bed, like Pulsatilla and Medorrhinum.

They can be practical people, able to do creative yet practical tasks with some inventiveness.

They are redfaced (reflecting an inner anger unknown to them), tend to heavy drinking, have great energy and big appetites, are extrovert and generous, giving in order to seek recognition, their posture for attracting love. They learnt in childhood that doing something was the main way of gaining appreciation and love, so it became a way of life. They can have a naive 'me first' approach, which is a bit clumsy socially.

They can be service engineers, surgeons on remote islands, plumbers, carpenters, or practical helpers. The less practical types can be deep philosophical thinkers, good on ideas but less good at doing and without much energy. They can be professors, inventive engineers, creative physics teachers, philosophical psychologists and New Age types. They will invent perpetual motion machines, antigravity machines, bicycles looking like Heath Robinson contraptions, anything that is weird, unusual and gets them noticed.

They relate better to ideas and theories than to their families. They think they are more intellectual than others, and look with disgust at lesser mortals.

This type can be tall, stooped, scientific, sloppy, unwashed and live in a tip, wear open sandals in winter and dirty clothes, and smell. Self-centred activity suits them. Inventing things or, more likely, having ideas that never materialize, is typical. They may be dope smokers, hopeful dreamers, lazy students, exaggerators.

The Sulphur woman can be a bit masculine and scathing with a quick wit and lots of brain power, and may be the practical one of the partnership.

In lectures and classrooms they are easy to spot. They stand up and ask interesting but basically theoretical questions while wearing eccentric 'notice me' clothing. If you joke about the theories it makes no difference; being self-absorbed they will not understand and will just ask another question.

As children they take everything apart to find out how it works and put it together again. They do not want to go to bed and miss out on interesting conversations. They are dirty children, into everything, nosy, bragging and self-centred.

Keynotes

Self-centred, egotistical, conceited. Inventive and creative. Children who are mechanically minded and always look dirty.

Full of theories. Very hot people, but can be cold. Itching and eczema. Collect 'useful things'.

Bite nails. Like meat fat, sweets, salt, spicy food and may not eat eggs. Untidy, with philosophical interests.

Trauma as disease

Mostly skin problems; they are the world's greatest itchers. Eczema.

A strong caution. If the person has got rid of most of their skin eruptions by creams such as cortisone, do not give Sulphur rashly. You could ask them to stop all creams and see what happens. If you stop the creams and *immediately* start treatment they may well break out all over, worse than they have ever been, and you will be blamed.

If you want to proceed in severe cases, go very gently. Get them to continue using the creams and when you see definite progress very slowly withdraw them. This applies especially to those with severe eruptions. In minor eruptions just proceed as normally instructed.

Another caution: *any* remedy can cure skin eruptions, so only use Sulphur if it fits.

Alcoholics with red noses. Piles.

TARANTULA

Keyword Speedy
Sources The poison of the spider

Stresses

Unrequited love. Bad news, scolding and punishment, even in the womb.

Working to tight deadlines. Excessive overwork; they work to hide from their inner emotional pain.

Punishment by a beating for failing an exam leading to the early onset of diabetes, for example.

Attitude

They are hyperactive, with very restless legs. They have the most messed up beds in the morning.

They are wound up like a tight spring, have superhuman stamina and strength when controlled. They are hurried in everything they do.

They are very hard working and competitive and can hold down two or three jobs and study for a higher degree and do exercise programmes every day. They especially like aerobics. They are very impatient with anyone slow.

Dancing wildly in circles is a sign, especially in extreme types. There is usually an aspect of going round in circles: in dancing, in gymnastics, in bed during sleep. They are very rhythmic. They must have music on to study. Rhythmic music calms them down. If they cannot dance then they might play the piano, knit or otherwise exercise their fingers. These are often busy.

They cannot bear red, green or black, and will not wear these colours or eat sweets of these colours.

They are cunning, devious and cagey, play tricks, feign illness and hide. Like the spider they spin a web that can be cunning, manipulative and sticky to envelop and trap you.

Sudden destructive behaviour may be followed by wild laughter. Hysteria can be calmed by music, or ends in laughter and apologies for their misbehaviour.

They have an aversion to touch and eat sand.

Trauma as disease

Intense sexuality, erotic mania, itching genitalia. Tumours of testes or ovaries. Backache, lumbago, sciatica.

Heart palpitation, angina pectoris and mitral valve disease. Chorea-like movements. Diabetes.

THUJA

Keywords   **The actor**
Source   **Pine tree bark**

Stresses

Guilt. Smallpox vaccination. Suppression of warts. Gonorrhoea in parents. Damp.

Attitude

Thuja types are secretive, guiltridden and deceitful. They are masqueraders with a sweet exterior, but they can be nasty underneath. They keep their true nature concealed in order not to arouse suspicion. They observe others but keep themselves secret.

They are self-satisfied and complacent, with a strange idea that there is something alive inside them or that they are fragile.

They need to be liked and yet they feel unlovable so they try to develop a persona that fits in and to imitate their chosen role model. They feel ugly inside but keep this secret and try hard to be liked.

They are neglected children. Symptoms occur especially at 3 a.m.

They have dreams of falling from a height, are worse in wet weather and have a desire for onions yet are upset by them.

It is indicated for bad effects of smallpox vaccination. The vaccination was stopped around 1950 in western Europe and around 1972 in eastern Europe.

Trauma as disease

Ridged, corrugated, thickened, ugly and deformed nails. Headaches.

Growths of any kind, especially warts and especially large ones.

Erosion of cervix. Asthma often following Arsenicum. Worse from damp. Sweetish perspiration.

Catarrhs of all kinds – thrush, nasal, postnasal. Birthmarks.

TUBERCULINUM

Keywords **Bored traveller**
Source **Tuberculosis**

Stresses

A history of tuberculosis, indicated by lifelong chest complaints in one parent or one grandparent.

Attitude

They have a desire to travel and change their life. There is a romantic longing, an unbearable sense of being unfulfilled.

They frequently change job, house, partner, decor, car, in a constant battle against boredom.

They are extremely irritable in the morning on waking and destructive when frustrated, with destructive fantasies. They are extremely irritable, with mental retardation and even autism.

Children of two have trantrums and are difficult. They break your favourite things, are hyperactive and obstinate.

They fear dogs and are allergic to cats, but may still keep them. They grind their teeth and shriek during sleep. They are optimistic.

They are worse before storms and like to drive with the windows open. They are likely to have chest complaints, and children may roll their heads against the bed and bang them repeatedly.

Children have fine hair on the spine and blue whites to the eyes. They crave cold milk, although they are allergic to it, salt, fat and ice cream.

Here is a quote from Stuart Wilde's *The Secrets of Life*:

> I have travelled constantly all my life. Wanderlust must have been in my veins at birth. I don't know about you but I find I use places up. When you first go to a place it seems magical and interesting and everything is new and fresh and it exhilarates you. Then one morning you wake up and the cute little store on the corner is not cute and a cockroach walks across your plate at the little bistro you loved so much. All the people you see tell you all the things they told you last week and suddenly you realize that you've drained the place of the magic it held for you. At that point my mind begins a faint hum. It's unintelligible at first, but as I listen carefully I can hear it getting louder and louder and I realize it's saying to me, 'Airport! Airport! Airport!'

I think that sums up Tuberculinum perfectly!

Trauma as disease

Chest infections and even pneumonia in cases with a family history of tuberculosis. Many coughs, especially a hard, short, dry, shallow or constant cough. Thin, narrow chest.

Asthma, better in the open air and better driving with window open. Children who do not thrive, frequent chest complaints, colds, etc. Recurring, even unexplained, fevers, recurring diarrhoea.

Headache like an iron band around the head; can be periodic. Arthritis with joint pains that are worse from cold, wet weather, worse on rising, worse at night with restlessness, better from heat and from motion.

Any complaints with the above picture.

CHAPTER TEN

Recovery from emotional suffering: self-help guidelines

FOCUS

To release the energy stored in deep traumas, to 'cure' them, needs highly focused energetic attention and persistence. With a homoeopathic remedy acting as the focus, this can be relatively easy as the hardest part, maintaining the focus, is done for you. The remedies are fixed, profound, deep-acting, ancient energies for healing that stay focused if you apply them correctly.

What often happens in real life, however, is a temporary fix. If, for example, fear was paramount in a person but a sympathetic ear bridged the fear and helped release some grief, then the next situation of grief would merely aggravate the problem and a trauma could be revived. While release from grief may be useful and life-saving, the root of the problem must still be dealt with for true healing and health.

Focusing on the trauma requires the patient's own commitment to change and especially the maintenance of the focus on the underlying trauma and not its outer effects. This is one of the great strengths of the homoeopathic approach. It names the trauma, giving it a homoeopathic remedy. It then addresses it in a focused way, persistently, even relentlessly, yet gently, at a pace entirely set by the patient themselves so that the old energy pattern is released until it resolves and dissolves, thus effecting healing.

PRESCRIBING AND WAITING

This process requires the correct remedy, or remedy sequence in some cases, and the persistence to keep on with it month in, month out, not necessarily taking the remedy all the time, until there is a real substantial change that is maintained without any further treatment. This can take years, after just one dose acts to start the cure, or a dose may be needed every few months.

The homoeopathic remedy will stimulate a curative response, quickly or slowly according to the vitality of the patient, and many factors will influence this. Younger people will generally be cured much faster than older ones. At ten it may take weeks, at forty months and at seventy even longer.

IT IS SAFE TO GET IT WRONG

Homoeopathy is very benign and user-friendly and if you follow the guidelines little can go wrong. Even if something does, stopping the remedy will soon alleviate the situation. It is very difficult to do harm with homoeopathic remedies if you act sensibly.

One major caution. Do not use combinations of remedies at the same time. They are not like vitamins, tonics, flower remedies or other medicaments of that kind. This is a profound system of in-depth curing and should be treated as such. The combination route can be both dangerous and suppressive. Only one remedy can be right at one time; the rest *must* be wrong. That is a serious warning.

You may, however, use one remedy after another; indeed this may be essential. By this I mean that you may select one remedy, use it for weeks or more likely months, perhaps even years, then change as the person changes. Children change and progress much faster than adults.

CURING GUIDELINES

There are two very separate skills here. The first is selecting your remedy, as we have discussed. The second is monitoring the curative process, so that the correct quantity and repetition are used. This is not difficult because it is often easy to monitor and because overdosing does not seem to matter, as the body does not notice excess stimulus much of the time. There are, however, sensitive people who know from experience that they over-react, and there is a specific way to prescribe for them (see page 227).

Signs of cure

Cure is indicated generally by combinations of the following responses.

1. Feeling better in yourself. Somehow you feel right, like your old self. Your spirit has come back, you are more confident. Feelings like this are a sure sign.
2. Being able to deal with life more effectively with less stress.
3. Having more energy, feeling more lively, able to do more, able to run again, laughing a lot.
4. Changing your life, even if it just seems to happen coincidentally. Perhaps your job changes or there is a shift in your attitude to work or study, or to colleagues, friends or family. Or you may have a more outgoing approach to life, changing your friendships somewhat, getting rid of bad relationships and taking on new ones.
5. Becoming more creative.
6. The homoeopathic aggravation. After taking a homoeopathic remedy there can be what is termed an aggravation, although with the remedies recommended here this is limited. The original trauma will not generally come back in anything like the intensity of the initial experience during healing unless it was very recent and very intense, when it may be desirable to consult someone skilled at listening. Usually, however, a spouse, parent or friend is all that is needed; Indeed, they may be the best people.
   A physical aggravation often occurs. This means becoming worse initially – perhaps for days, weeks or even months if the physical symptoms have been around a

long time. Generally speaking, the worsening is either short and painful or slow, less dramatic and more drawn out.

This worsening is often based on toxins being eliminated through the outlets of the body, via the stool or urine, through the skin as rashes, pimples, boils or fever, through the nose as sneezing, a cold, etc., or through the mouth by vomiting. Boils often occur near toxic sites. The recovery stage is generally as long as the worsening stage, so if you have a one-day aggravation, the next day it may go. Temporary worsening of symptoms is not then to be interpreted as side effects but as signs of your body working to heal itself.

7. Having a brief temporary return of old symptoms is good, especially when they return in reverse sequence to the original occurrence. These may be transitory – just a few seconds like a flashback – or longer-lasting like a cloud passing. This is called the law of cure and happens occasionally.

   The law of cure also means that symptoms will be eliminated in an order, from serious to less serious ones, from internal organs to external or less critical ones, from inside out as we say, and from above down. However, respiratory and heart improvements can go up and outwards as these go from the lungs (serious) to the throat and nose (less serious). The return of a cough in asthma can be a good sign that the chest is having a clear-out.

   So asthma becoming a skin rash or sneezing bouts is good; but hayfever or eczema becoming asthma is not cure, it is suppression and wrong.

8. It is fine if physical symptoms just get better, provided the process fits the law of cure.

9. Occasionally a meaningful dream or sequence of dreams, even if it is not understood, could be a healing indication if the dream *feels* right, important or positive in some way. For example, if the trauma was to do with grief, seeing the dead person in a dream in a nice way would be good. For fear, feeling a deep release in a dream would be good. Trust the *feeling* of the dream experience.

10. Generally the sequence is that you first start to feel better

mentally and then your physical symptoms may temporarily worsen as the toxins eliminate. A light diet or a fruit fast may reduce these effects if they are strong.

If previous physical symptoms were spasmodic, as in asthma or headaches, they will die out, subsequent attacks becoming less severe, of shorter duration and less frequent. Milder recurrences are not, then, a time to panic and represcribe once a cure has been started.

Signs of non-cure

These are the most obvious:

1. No effect – wrong remedy.
2. A new symptom – definitely wrong remedy.
3. Reverse law of cure, suppression – stop, wait, with antidote if necessary.
4. Aggravation without later benefit – close but wrong remedy.

THE INNER HEALING PROCESS

Traumas are held in flesh, cells, muscles, tendons, posture, organs, memories, and as old emotions and limiting thoughts. As the remedy works away at stimulating the immune system, the tensions, distortions and memories are gradually released so that all the energy used to hold these in is freed and flows again in the body, providing more energy for living. Also as the energy flows, old feelings of hurt dissipate and the soul finds more clarity, which we experience as feeling like our old selves again or being at peace within, or something similar.

We may respond differently to old situations, not out of the old pattern of thought or feeling but in a new way; or we may seize upon opportunities we previously let go. In this way real changes come about.

Likewise as the energy is released, the blockages disperse and emotional knots are untied, the consequential tension in the muscles of the back or around the joint relaxes. Or the anger held in the womb disperses and back comes the sexual urge again. Or the fear of attack is resolved in dreams and trembling while talking and the fear of walking alone dissolve. With grief, frequently some small event will trigger deep unexpected crying for someone who may have died years ago; it is as if it has just happened and then you get over it.

All these emotional releases are possible in response to some apparently small event, causing a deep release of old trauma. But often nothing specific is noticed, just an improvement. This may be the situation for a majority of people. If you do not normally notice your feelings strongly, then recovery will be similar, as the healing process is in essence hidden from view and can often pass unnoticed.

REMEDIES AND PRESCRIBING GUIDELINES

Remedies

The remedies used here are very similar to the ones you can buy at most healthfood shops but they are prepared slightly differently. Ideally, buy the required remedy in LM1 potency from one of the listed homoeopathic pharmacies. See the ordering information and pharmacy list for the exact specification. If you can only get the 6th, 6x or 3c, 6c or 9c potency in a bottle of tablets from the local chemist, use one crushed pill from this as the seed granule for the glass bottle described below. It is not important whether it dissolves or not.

If you have a liquid remedy in a bottle sent to you from a homoeopathic chemist, then proceed to step 1 below, but if you order the remedy in LM1 granules then get a 100 ml glass bottle from any local chemist, fill it two thirds full with pure (distilled) water from the chemist and put in just one tiny seed granule (or one crushed tablet). It is very tiny but that is all that is needed. LM1 granules are very small and a vial should last a lifetime.

Step 1   Taking the remedy

Each day follow the procedure as below.

1. Bang the bottle containing the remedy seed ten times on a solid surface that will not break the bottle such as a book or a carpet.
2. Then put half a teaspoonful from the bottle into half a glass of water; exact quantities are unimportant.
3. Stir vigorously.
4. Take a teaspoonful in the mouth and hold it there a few seconds (with children, just put it in the mouth). The liquid will disperse of its own accord.
5. Throw the rest of the contents away.

Each day repeat the whole process.

Step 2   Monitoring progress

The golden rule is that you take or give the remedy until it acts and then *stop*. If you get any reaction, whether 'good' or 'bad', stop. Reactions are given in 'signs of cure' above and briefly these are:

- you feel better;
- you have noticeably more energy;
- the symptoms get better;
- the symptoms get worse;
- old symptoms come back strongly;
- old symptoms from years back return briefly;
- symptoms return according to the law of cure;
- toxins are eliminated from the body by pimples, rashes, boils, fevers, vomiting or changes in stool or urine;
- any combination of the above; the more that occur the more certain it is that cure is happening and the more reason to *stop*.

If you notice nothing much, continue until you have a definite improvement that you are sure about. Then *stop*. If nothing happens after two weeks the remedy is probably wrongly selected. If you are sure it is right but there is little to show for it, persist for up to two months before giving up.

People often cannot really believe that it is happening and are reluctant to stop at the first solid sign of cure. But you can and *it is a good idea to do so*. The cure will then proceed under its own momentum; like a stone rolling down hill, once it is going there is no point chasing it to kick it harder.

Once you have stopped, wait. Let the cure proceed under its own steam. Even if later you are sure things are getting worse again, if there is a possible temporary cause for the relapse, like a cold, stress, a visit to the dentist or a period, wait and see if recovery resumes by itself. It should and often will. The basic rule is do not represcribe on the first relapse; it will often pass. Just wait and see.

Three-glass method

This may be needed, for an old person, where a strong reaction is inadvisable, in a feeble child, in an adult where the problem is deep or goes back generations, or sensitive people and those who over-react. But these cases should preferably be referred to a professional homoeopath.

Proceed as in Step 1 above but with three half-full glasses of water. Put one teaspoonful from the first glass into the second, stir vigorously, put one teaspoonful from the second glass into the third, stir and take one teaspoonful from the third glass. Then throw the contents of all the glasses away.

Very feeble old people can omit banging the bottle.

Precautions for patients

Do not clean your teeth with toothpaste fifteen minutes before or after taking the remedy.

As far as practical, do not eat or drink for fifteen minutes before and after taking the remedy. However, it is best to take it rather than to skip it if you are pressed for time.

It is best not to drink real coffee during treatment, nor ideally for three months after treatment; decaffeinated coffee is fine and so is tea.

Alcohol is all right except in the case of some problems which are related to it, such as psoriasis.

The contraceptive pill and prescribed drugs can slow or stop progress or restrict it.

Refilling the bottle

If the bottle is nearly empty, with half an inch or so left, just refill it two thirds with pure water, bang it forty times on the solid surface and continue as before. Do not worry, less is more in homoeopathy. This is also better than buying a new bottle of LM1, which will have a lower potency than your original bottle after all the banging.

Repeating

If you are sure you need more, repeat steps 1 and 2 again. There is great scope for error here, however. Repeating too soon is a common problem, as almost everyone seems to think that more is better. Always err on the side of caution in an apparent relapse after a good curative response. Waiting is the name of the game. Any relapse after a stressful event is likely to pass. Wait and only repeat if the old situation is definitely recurring pretty much as it was.

If, however, the picture has changed, then the original remedy may not be indicated (but this is unlikely in many cases); you will have to select a new remedy if this new state persists.

Persistence

Slow, steady, considered, monitored, persistent use of the remedy when it is called for is the main task once it is shown to work. The less it is used the better.

The cure may take a day, a week, a month or a year or more, and the deeper the trauma or the longer the family history of trauma, the longer the cure. Some cures will be very quick; even after the very first dose there will be remarkable effects. More often, the cure will be by occasional doses at long intervals over many years. This is fine. You may find that after a week or two you just take the remedy when you really fell you need it. It often seems to happen naturally. Obviously the total cure takes much longer than the time over which you take the remedy. The remedy is only the catalyst, it only acts for a few seconds. Vital energy changes fast. Once it has acted the cure goes on inside for weeks, months or years without further stimulus. Nature takes a while to sort itself out.

Record what you do

Make sure you make notes about what you do. Good records may save the day if you become confused or uncertain. Have a special note book for this.

A stronger dose?

If when repeating the remedy it gradually fails to work, these are the most likely reasons:

1. The remedy was wrong to start with and the cure is only superficial. If this seems likely, reconsider the original facts and any others that you have since learnt and try again with a more suitable remedy.
2. The person may have shifted to another trauma, or trauma layer in the case of a multiple trauma, and this now has to be addressed.
3. If the cure was definite and certain yet there is now a relapse and the same picture is occurring as before, then other possibilities are likely. The remedy may need strengthening, but this is unlikely. More likely causes are: a block to letting go, some maintaining cause such as a difficult life situation; a body poisoning like coffee counteracting the remedy; medical drugs undermining the remedy action; or an undermining disease from the past, such as tuberculosis in a parent. A disease history block will require a homoeopath.

If the remedy does need strengthening this is how to go about it. Turn the bottle upside down, drain it and the cap for five minutes on a tissue, then refill it two thirds full with pure water and bang it forty times. This will dilute and strengthen it, using the residue liquid on the inside of the bottle.

Mistakes

The most common prescribing mistakes are as follows:

1. Wrong remedy. Usually nothing much happens, but it might act superficially for a while.
2. Not appreciating that a cure is taking place. It is usually better to have someone helping you because they can be more objective.
3. Repeating in panic and too often (through the belief that more is better, a cultural norm, but one you must reverse).

Storage

If a remedy in a bottle is to be stored for a long time, put it in the fridge. The granules or pills will last a hundred years or more if kept in a non-smelly place in a sealed container. Samuel Hahnemann's remedies still work after nearly 200 years; there is no limit to the shelf life of homoeopathic remedies.

Examples of prescribing

Causation   Grief from death of father five years ago.
Problem   Sleeplessness.
Remedy chosen   Ignatia.
Dose   Ignatia LM1 daily.
Effect   After one dose felt weepy then slept for twelve hours, which was very unusual, and felt different. Stopped as the remedy was definitely acting. No repeats ever needed.

Causation   Death of father and mother, and divorce.
Problem   Headaches.
Remedy chosen   Nat mur.

Dose   Nat mur LM1 daily.
Effect   Taken daily for two weeks when gradually headaches seemed to be much better. Stopped. After six weeks they returned after a period. Waited; they went away again without help. After another four weeks they started to come back as before. Repeated remedy for three days, till they stopped again. Used in tailing off sequence as needed.

Causation   Unknown, early parenting effects.
Problem   Itchy rash on chest.
Remedy chosen   Sulphur.
Dose   Sulphur LM1 daily (see precautions for skin in Sulphur pattern).
Effect   Gradual improvement over two weeks, 75 per cent better, better sleeping too. Dose Sulphur LM1 three times a week, reducing to a maintaining dose when minor outbreaks occur.

Causation   Isolation experiences around birth. Three weeks in an incubator.
Problem   Bouts of deep depression, loss of creativity. Sleeplessness.
Remedy chosen   Aurum.
Dose   Aurum LM1 daily.
Effect   Within weeks a return to her old spirit, becoming creatively productive again, and no depressive bouts. Repeated only as needed, about every two or three months.

CHAPTER ELEVEN

Final comments

In this book I have looked at the world through a lens called trauma and suffering. I have shown that suffering permeates the whole human family, at all levels of society, in all countries, races, professions and activities. I hope I have shown that trauma and suffering underlie much if not all of human malfunction and are the basis from which most forms of acute and chronic disease emanate. I believe I have shown that our institutions — home, school, hospitals, prisons, armies, politicians, etc. — are acting out suffering and are badly distorted by it.

This may seem like a narrow view, but it is how I have experienced the last two decades of helping people. It is built upon a long sustained tradition and the support of many colleagues. Because I am involved in training courses for hundreds of doctors, I know from their feedback that I am not exaggerating the medical problems.

In patients from all walks of life, I have witnessed the transformation of consciousness, from suffering and disease to freedom, vitality and happiness.

There is a way of changing this situation of universal suffering that would be incredibly effective, easy to implement at very low costs and very safe in sensible hands. It is, of course, homoeopathic medicine. But it is currently a very slow process, so I hope this book will bridge the gap while you are waiting.

There are, of course, many other wonderful movements and healing systems that are doing similar work, spreading the word and helping to transform society right now. I have experienced many forms of alternative medicine — meditation, psychotherapy, shamanism, etc. — and as I see it pluralism is the way forward in all walks of life, including medicine.

But I wish to stress that, beyond all this, the power of homoeopathic remedies applied by correct principles and methods is unique, and the world has yet to appreciate it fully. There is nothing else in my experience that can act so deeply and effectively.

Appendix
Further information

BOOKS AND ARTICLES

Homoeopathy has a 200-year-history which has created a tremendous wealth of information, much of it wonderful, a lot of it confusing and a lot totally out of date. Most of it was written in the last century or is current but written as if the authors were in the last century. Precious little relates to our time. However, this situation is being remedied. Here are the ones I recommend.

The best homoeopathic books

All three are expensive but better than most of the rest. With these three you have high-quality information.

Synoptic Materia Medica, Frans Vermeulen, Merlin Publishers, Netherlands, 1993. Gives very good trauma pictures.

Materia Medica, Roger Morrison, Hahnemann Clinic Publishing, Albany, California, 1993. Very good people pictures, the best so far.

The Homoeopathic Treatment of Children, Paul Herscu, North Atlantic Books, Berkeley, California, 1991.

Other homoeopathic books

Portraits of Homoeopathic Medicines, Vols. 1, 2 and 3, Catherine Coulter, North Atlantic Books, Berkeley, California, 1987–9.

Essence of Materia Medica, George Vithoulkas, Jain Publishers, New Delhi, 1988.

Homoeopathy, Medicine for the New Man, George Vithoulkas, Arco, New York, 1979. A good introductory read.

The Science of Homoeopathy, George Vithoulkas, Thorsons, London, 1993. The first half of this book could be called the 'science of health'. By a leading world health creator and thinker.

A Homoeopathic Love Story, Rima Handley, North Atlantic Books, Berkeley, 1990. An account of Samuel Hahnemann in a beautifully written book.

Homoeopathic Pharmacopoeia, M Bhattacharyya and Co., Homoeopathic Chemists, 73 Netaji Subhas Rd, Calcutta 1, 1980. For those who want to make their own remedies, this is the cheapest available book.

Warning

Almost all homoeopathic books will tend to talk about homoeopathic potency in a different way from this book and you may find this confusing. If you stick to the information in this book, you will do well. After fifteen years my conclusion is that homoeopathic potency is mostly dogma, based on nothing more than prejudice – nothing measurable by anything objective. The subject drives more students of homoeopathy to despair than any other. The system I advocate in this book is based on the final realizations of Samuel Hahnemann, the last gem of his life's work, which, because of an historical accident, was not introduced into general use until very recently, after a lot of other methods became standard.

Homoeopathic research

M. A. Taylor and D.T. Reilly. 'Is homoeopathy a placebo effect? Hay fever trial'. *The Lancet*, 1986, 2 (8512), 881–6.
David Reilly has completed several research experiments on homoeopathy and featured in several BBC TV programmes.

J. Benveniste. 'Human basophil degranulation triggered by very dilute antiserum against IgE'. *Nature*, 1988, 333, 816–18.
Showed conclusively that potency 200 can be detected yet it is a dilution of 10^{-400}!

Dr Peter Fisher *et al.* 'Fibrositis'. *British Medical Journal*, 1989, 299, 365–6.

Books about trauma

Making Sense of Suffering, K. Conrad Stettbecker, Penguin, Harmondworth, 1991. The first half of this book is excellent.

The Human Side of Human Beings, Harvey Jackins, Rational Island Publishers, Seattle, 1972. Old but clear, simple and profound.
Both describe the wounding process in detail.

Psyche and Substance, Edward Whitmont, North Atlantic Books, Berkeley, California, 1980. Refers to psychology and homoeopathy.

For parents and parents-to-be

The Continuum Concept, Jean Liedloff, Penguin, Harmondworth, 1989. Explains separation wounding as no one else has. Essential reading for parents-to-be.

For Your Own Good (1987) and *Drama of Being a Child* (1974), Alice Miller, Virago, London. Examine the effects of parenting and abuse. A *must* for parents.

The Immunization Decision, R. Neustaedtr, North Atlantic Books, Berkeley, California, 1990.

General books

The Secrets of Life, Stuart Wilde, White Dove International Inc, Taos, New Mexico, 1991. A real gem.

Confessions of a Medical Heretic, R. Mendelssohn, Warner Books, London, 1979. A doctor's view of medicine as practised today.

How to Be a Healthy Patient, Stephen Fulder, Hodder and Stoughton, Sevenoaks, 1991. Tells you how to cross-question a consultant and win!

Families and How to Survive Them, Robin Skynner and John Cleese, Methuen, London, 1983.

The New People Making, Virginia Satir, Science and Behaviour Books Inc, USA, 1989. An all-time 'bible'.

Homoeopathic first aid and use in the home

Complete Handbook of Homoeopathy, Miranda Castro, Macmillan, Basingstoke, 1989.

Everybody's Guide to Homoeopathic Medicines, Stephen Cummings and Dana Ullman, Gollancz, London, 1990. The best all-round introduction and family guide.

Homoeopathic Medicine at Home, M. Panos and J. Hiemlich, Corgi, London, 1980. A good first aid and self-help book.

Homoeopathic Cures for Common Diseases, Dr Yudhvir Singh, Orient Paperbacks, New Delhi, 1988. Useful for travellers for infectious diseases.

SUPPORT AGENCIES

If you find you have problems that this book has highlighted but you do not feel able to use it to help yourself, then there are many sources of help.

Obviously in some places doctors may be able to refer you or help you. Therapists of any holistic persuasion may be the first place to turn. Acupuncture, psychotherapy and counselling would be obvious sources of help if homoeopathy is not available. First ask friends if they can recommend someone or check with an organization of repute. Or just ask a few local therapists by telephone if they think they can help you with your problems and see which response you prefer. Healers exist in many countries and can be very good; herbalists or phytotherapists likewise. The quality of the person is usually more important than the therapy practised.

HOMOEOPATHIC BOOK AND INFORMATION SUPPLIERS

Homoeopathic booksellers in the UK include Minerva Books, 6 Bothwell Street, London W6 8DY. Tel: 071 385 1361.

The Complete Repertory and MacRepertory, computerized homoeopathic information, materia medica and repertory, are essential tools for professional homoeopaths and are available from The Homoeopathic Bicycle Co, 16 St Michael Mount, Northampton NN1 4JG, tel: 0604 28768, who will also advise you of

European suppliers. In the USA, phone 0101 415 457 0678 or fax 0101 415 457 0688.

PHARMACIES

UK

Helios Homoeopathic Pharmacy, 97 Camden Road, Tunbridge Wells, Kent TN1 1QR. Tel: 0892 536393.
Ainsworth Homoeopathic Pharmacy, 38 New Cavendish Street, London W1M 7LH. Tel: 071 487 5253.
Nelson's Homoeopathic Pharmacy, 73 Duke Street, London W1M 6BY. Tel: 071 629 3118.
Galen Homoeopathic Pharmacy, Lewel, Dorchester, Dorset. Tel: 0305 263996.
Buxton and Grant, 176 Whiteladies Road, Bristol BS8 2XU. Tel: 0272 735025.
Freeman's, 7 Eaglesham Road, Clarkston, Glasgow G76 7BU. Tel: 041 644 1165.

Overseas

Boericke and Tafel Inc, 1011 Arch St, Philadelphia PA 19107, USA. Tel: 215 922 2967.
Martin and Pleasance, PO Box 4, Collingwood, Victoria 3066, Australia. Tel: 61341 99733.
Bhandari Homoeopathic Stores, Opp York Hotel, Conn Circus, New Delhi. Tel: 320560.

There are homoeopathic pharmacies in the main cities of many countries.

SUPPLIES

The Homoeopathic Supply Company has many accessories, including plastic envelopes, kit boxes, phials, etc. The address is: 4 Nelson Road, Sheringham, Norfolk NR26 8BU. Tel: 0263 824683.

Most UK chemists stock the 6c potency of most of the remedies used in this book. But do not assume that the average chemist knows anything about the remedies at all. Their advice is likely to be based on extremely limited knowledge and false information. Take no notice of it.

FINDING HOMOEOPATHS

The Society of Homoeopaths in the UK (address as below) publish a reliable register.

There is often a problem in identifying homoeopaths who work holistically and classically – the approach I have outlined in this book – so here are some questions to ask to ensure that you find one.

First ask simply what sort of homoeopath they are. 'Classical' is what you want to hear. 'I do what seems appropriate' means something else and they are probably dodging the issue. Ask too if they practise anything else; if so it is usually a bad sign.

Ask if they use one remedy at a time or combinations of remedies. Combinations means you should go elsewhere.

Ask if they use any machines in diagnosis and remedy. These are bad signs. Ask if they use dowsing. My experience is that such people are often inaccurate, although there are some notable exceptions. (Healers using pendulums may, however, be excellent and so in fact are a few homoeopaths, but not many.)

If you discover that they practise conventional medicine and homoeopathy together then they are probably not classical or they lack ability.

If they say they are 'unicists', meaning one remedy at a time, that is the term used for classical in eastern Europe.

If they prescribe combinations of homoeopathic remedies, this is not homoeopathy at all but conventional medicine using homoeopathic remedies in a potentially suppressive way. If they use just one remedy at a time and one dose then they are probably classical.

Reference sources for homoeopaths

In the UK, the Society of Homoeopaths. Send a stamped addressed envelope to them at 2 Artisan Road, Northampton, NN1 4HU. Tel: 0604 21400.

In the USA, Homoeopathic Education Services, 2124 Kitteredge Street, Berkeley, California 94704. Tel: 510 649 0294, fax: 510 649 1955. Also for training, research and homoeopathic contacts.

Homoeopathic pharmacies can usually give you information.

TRAINING IN HOMOEOPATHY

At a first aid level you should ask your local homoeopath who may be willing to train you. Booksellers sell first aid charts and homoeopathic chemists remedies and creams.

For professional training in Britain there are many options. I teach for the London College of Classical Homoeopathy, at Morley College, 61 Westminster Bridge Rd, London SE1 7HG, which currently runs the only full-time training in classical homoeopathy, and part-time courses in London, Edinburgh, Sofia, Bucharest, Budapest, Prague, Brno, Bratislava and elsewhere.

The Society of Homoeopaths has a list of all the UK colleges of homoeopathy, but ask for the list of classical colleges, as some are not.

There is also a correspondence course that is very good. It is available from the School of Homoeopathy (contactable through the Society of Homoeopaths), and may be regarded as a first step to professional training.

AND FINALLY AN APPEAL

Many of the stories of suffering in this book come from areas of the world where poverty is the norm. Along with a dedicated unpaid team of colleagues, I spend most of my time teaching in such countries and creating new seminar programmes to train doctors and healers in homoeopathy.

Funds for this activity are very limited and much that could be done is not being done for the lack of relatively small amounts of money.

If you would like to help with this project you could donate directly to the Homoeopathy Trust, a charity which helps to fund it when it has resources to do so, specifying that your donation is for this purpose. For donations and for details of training programmes please write directly to the London College of Classical Homoeopathy, Morley College, 61 Westminster Bridge Rd, London, SE1 7HG, or to me at Morley College. (The author is not available for postal consultations.)

Index